Contemporary Controversies in Foot and Ankle Surgery

Guest Editor

NEAL M. BLITZ, DPM

CLINICS IN PODIATRIC MEDICINE AND SURGERY

www.podiatric.theclinics.com

Consulting Editor
THOMAS ZGONIS, DPM, FACFAS

July 2012 • Volume 29 • Number 3

SAUNDERS an imprint of ELSEVIER, Inc.

W.B. SAUNDERS COMPANY
A Division of Elsevier Inc.

1600 John F. Kennedy Boulevard • Suite 1800 • Philadelphia, Pennsylvania 19103-2899

http://www.theclinics.com

CLINICS IN PODIATRIC MEDICINE AND SURGERY Volume 29, Number 3
July 2012 ISSN 0891-8422, ISBN-13: 978-1-4557-4943-0

Editor: Patrick Manley

Clinics in Podiatric Medicine and Surgery (ISSN 0891-8422) is published quarterly by Elsevier Inc., 360 Park Avenue South, New York, NY 10010-1710. Months of issue are January, April, July, and October. Business and Editorial Offices: 1600 John F. Kennedy Blvd., Ste. 1800, Philadelphia, PA 19103-2899. Customer Service Office: 3251 Riverport Lane, Maryland Heights, MO 63043. Periodicals postage paid at New York, NY and additional mailing offices. Subscription prices are $292.00 per year for US individuals, $410.00 per year for US institutions, $148.00 per year for US students and residents, $350.00 per year for Canadian individuals, $508.00 for Canadian institutions, $415.00 for international individuals, $508.00 per year for international institutions and $208.00 per year for Canadian and foreign students/residents. To receive student/resident rate, orders must be accompanied by name of affiliated institution, date of term, and the *signature* of program/residency coordinator on institution letterhead. Orders will be billed at individual rate until proof of status is received. Foreign air speed delivery is included in all *Clinics* subscription prices. All prices are subject to change without notice. POSTMASTER: Send address changes to *Clinics in Podiatric Medicine and Surgery*, Elsevier Health Sciences Division, Subscription Customer Service, 3251 Riverport Lane, Maryland Heights, MO 63043. **Customer Service: 1-800-654-2452 (US). From outside of the US, call 314-447-8871. Fax: 314-447-8029. E-mail: JournalsCustomerService-usa@elsevier.com (for print support); JournalsOnlineSupport-usa@elsevier.com (for online support).**

Reprints. For copies of 100 or more of articles in this publication, please contact the Commercial Reprints Department, Elsevier Inc., 360 Park Avenue South, New York, NY 10010-1710. Tel.: 212-633-3812; Fax: 212-462-1935; E-mail: reprints@elsevier.com.

Clinics in Podiatric Medicine and Surgery is covered in *MEDLINE/PubMed (Index Medicus)* and *EMBASE/Excerpta Medica.*

Printed and bound by CPI Group (UK) Ltd, Croydon, CR0 4YY

Transferred to Digital Print 2012

CLINICS IN PODIATRIC MEDICINE AND SURGERY

CONSULTING EDITOR
THOMAS ZGONIS, DPM, FACFAS

Contributors

CONSULTING EDITOR

THOMAS ZGONIS, DPM, FACFAS
Director, Podiatric Surgical Residency and Reconstructive Fellowship Programs; Chief, Division of Podiatric Medicine and Surgery; Associate Professor, Department of Orthopedic Surgery, The University of Texas Health Science Center at San Antonio, San Antonio, Texas

GUEST EDITOR

NEAL M. BLITZ, DPM, FACFAS
Chief of Foot Surgery, Associate Chairman of Orthopaedics, Department of Orthopaedics Surgery, Bronx-Lebanon Hospital Center, Albert Einstein College of Medicine, Bronx, New York

AUTHORS

RONALD BELIN, DPM
Broadlawns Medical Center, Des Moines, Iowa

NICHOLAS J. BEVILACQUA, DPM, FACFAS
North Jersey Orthopaedic Specialists, PA, Teaneck, New Jersey

NEAL M. BLITZ, DPM, FACFAS
Chief of Foot Surgery, Associate Chairman of Orthopaedics, Department of Orthopaedics Surgery, Bronx-Lebanon Hospital Center, Albert Einstein College of Medicine, Bronx, New York

CLAIRE M. CAPOBIANCO, DPM, AACFAS
Private Practice, Orthopaedic Associates of Southern Delaware, Lewes, Delaware

SCOTT CARRINGTON, BA
Des Moines University College of Podiatric Medicine and Surgery, Des Moines, Iowa

J. DANNY CHOUNG, DPM
Chief, Department of Podiatric Surgery, Kaiser Foundation Hospital, San Rafael, California

LAWRENCE A. DIDOMENICO, DPM
Section Chief of Podiatry, St. Elizabeth's Hospital; Adjunct Professor, Ohio College of Podiatric Medicine; Director of Reconstructive Rearfoot and Ankle Surgical Fellowship, Ankle and Foot Care Centers, Ohio College of Podiatric Medicine, Youngstown, Ohio

NIK GATALYAK, DPM
Fellow, Reconstructive Rearfoot and Ankle Surgical Fellowship, Ankle and Foot Care Centers, Ohio College of Podiatric Medicine, Youngstown, Ohio

ROBERT M. GREENHAGEN, DPM
Private Practice, Foot and Ankle Center of Nebraska, Omaha, Nebraska

GRAHAM A. HAMILTON, DPM, FACFAS
Department of Orthopedics and Podiatric Surgery, Kaiser Permanente Medical Center, Antioch, California

ADAM R. JOHNSON, DPM
Department of Surgery, Hennepin County Medical Center, Minneapolis, Minnesota

KLAUS J. KERNBACH, DPM, FACFAS
Attending Podiatric Surgeon and Research Director, Kaiser North Bay Consortium Residency Program, Department of Podiatry, Kaiser Foundation Hospital, Vallejo, California

RUTH A. PEACE, DPM
Kaiser San Francisco Bay Area Foot and Ankle Residency Program, Kaiser Foundation Hospital, Oakland, California

JOHN J. STAPLETON, DPM, FACFAS
Associate, Foot and Ankle Surgery, VSAS Orthopaedics; Chief of Podiatric Surgery, Lehigh Valley Hospital, Allentown; Clinical Assistant Professor of Surgery, Penn State College of Medicine, Hershey, Pennsylvania

CRYSTAL L. RAMANUJAM, DPM, MSc
Assistant Professor, Division of Podiatric Medicine and Surgery, Department of Orthopaedic Surgery, The University of Texas Health Science Center at San Antonio, San Antonio, Texas

MHER VARTIVARIAN, DPM
Department of Podiatric Surgery, Kaiser Foundation Hospital, San Rafael, California

DAPHNE YEN-DOUANGMALA, DPM
Department of Podiatric Surgery, Kaiser Foundation Hospital, San Rafael, California

THOMAS ZGONIS, DPM, FACFAS
Director, Podiatric Surgical Residency and Reconstructive Fellowship Programs; Chief, Division of Podiatric Medicine and Surgery; Associate Professor, Department of Orthopedic Surgery, The University of Texas Health Science Center at San Antonio, San Antonio, Texas

Contents

End-stage arthritis of the first metatarsophalangeal joint (MTPJ) typically results in anexophytic process with marked limitation of motion. Pain may occur from the degenerative process itself and/or the bone spur formation that may become directly inflamed from shoe gear. The best surgical treatment for end-stage arthrosis of the big toe joint continues to be a controversial topic despite hallux rigidus being recognized clinically for more than 100 years. Although joint-sparing procedures are considered, arthrodesis is recommended, as this procedure is definitive and produces predictable results.

In cases of painful complex hammertoe deformity, there is no single approach that can be used in all circumstances. If conservative care fails, surgical management may include interphalangeal joint arthroplasty, arthrodesis, and/or plantar plate repair. The best and most pragmatic surgical plan must be patient-centered, taking the age, activity level, expectations of the patient, and precise etiology of the hammertoe deformity into account.

The Lapidus procedure should no longer be considered a strict nonweight-bearing bunionectomy. In the past few years, several studies have emerged demonstrating that early weightbearing after a Lapidus fusion is indeed possible with satisfactory fusion rates. This is mainly because of improved fixation techniques available today, which have allowed for better stabilization of the fusion site. Surgeons should still properly indicate patients for early weightbearing protocols.

Subtalar joint arthroereisis is a surgical procedure that addresses symptomatic flexible flatfoot deformities using an extraarticular implant within the sinus tarsi. Three groups of implants have been developed for this procedure: self-locking wedges, axis-altering devices, and impact-blocking devices. The self-locking wedge implants are the focus of this article, relative to its use, limitations, and controversies in the pediatric and adult population.

End-stage ankle arthritis is a debilitating condition that leads to pain and swelling in the ankle joint, with symptoms aggravated by standing and ambulation. Ankle arthritis commonly results from a history of trauma, or a series of recurrent injuries to the ankle. However, it may develop from other causes such as uneven loading of the ankle joint caused by an alignment deformity or from inflammatory arthritis such as rheumatoid arthritis, gout, or secondary to a serious joint infection. Patients with severe ankle arthritis often have limited ankle motion with an antalgic gait.

Contracture of the Achilles-gastrocnemius-soleus complex leading to ankle equinus has been linked to the development of various foot disorders. Decrease in ankle dorsiflexion results in an increase in plantar pressures and in diabetes and neuropathy, increased pressures can lead to ulceration and possibly the formation of Charcot foot. Surgical management of the equinus deformity corrects this abnormality and has the potential to avert the development of Charcot foot or ankle. Gastrocnemius recession, tendo-Achilles lengthening, and Achilles tenotomy have all been offered as surgical solutions to this condition. This article reviews ankle equinus and compares the treatment options available. A video of Hoke's triple hemisection has been included with this article and can be viewed at www.podiatric.theclinics.com.

Charcot neuroarthropathy of the foot and ankle is a devastating neuropathic complication that can eventually lead to a lower extremity amputation in the presence of an ulceration or infection. Current surgical approaches for the management of the diabetic Charcot foot and ankle deformities are largely based on expert opinions in various fixation methods attempting to avoid major postoperative complications. The goal of this article is to discuss the advantages and disadvantages of various internal, external, or combined fixation methods as they relate to the inherent challenges in the management of the diabetic Charcot foot.

A wide array of reconstructive options exists for soft tissue coverage of diabetic foot wounds; however, each case depends on the patient's medical comorbidities, wound type, anatomy of the affected site, and level of contamination. Although autologous skin grafts have traditionally played a pivotal role in the coverage of diabetic wounds, several advanced biological skin substitutes have become available, providing surgeons with additional choices in the management of these challenging wounds. This article reviews these surgical modalities by presenting indications for every option and clinical scenario that may benefit from their combined use.

Current Concepts and Techniques in Foot and Ankle Surgery

The second metatarsophalangeal joint is prone to specific and varied pathology that is well understood and may exist in isolation or in combination with other forefoot abnormality. Surgical treatment options for managing end-stage second metatarsophalangeal abnormalities have been minimally studied and exist primarily in case studies and series in the literature. As a result, surgical approaches remain controversial and warrant further discussion.

Puncture wounds of the foot are a common injury, and infection associated with these injuries may result in considerable morbidity. The pathophysiology and management of a puncture wound is dependent on the material that punctures the foot, the location and depth of the wound, time to presentation, footwear, and underlying health status of the patient. Puncture wounds should not be treated lightly, so accurate diagnosis, assessment, and treatment are paramount. Early incision and drainage, vaccination, and the use of proper antibiotics can lead to positive outcomes and prevent limb-threatening circumstances.

CLINICS IN PODIATRIC MEDICINE AND SURGERY

FORTHCOMING ISSUES

October 2012
Ankle Arthritis
Jesse B. Burks, DPM, *Guest Editor*

January 2013
Primary Total Ankle Replacement
Thomas S. Roukis, DPM, *Guest Editor*

April 2013
Revision Total Ankle Replacement
Thomas S. Roukis, DPM, *Guest Editor*

RECENT ISSUES

April 2012
Foot and Ankle Trauma
Denise Mandi, DPM, *Guest Editor*

January 2012
Arthrodesis of the Foot and Ankle
Steven F. Boc, DPM and
Vincent Muscarella, DPM, *Guest Editors*

October 2011
Advances in Fixation Technology for the Foot and Ankle
Patrick R. Burns, DPM, *Guest Editor*

Foreword

Contemporary Controversies in Foot and Ankle Surgery

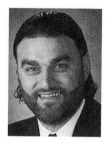

Thomas Zgonis, DPM
Consulting Editor

This edition of *Clinics in Podiatric Medicine and Surgery* brings together some of the most popular controversies in foot and ankle surgery. A variety of topics in elective, reconstructive, and trauma surgery are well covered by contemplating the procedures selected with each condition. Treatment options for the end-stage hallux rigidus, digital deformity, Lapidus arthrodesis, and subtalar joint arthroereisis are debated with the most recent advances in technology. Primary arthrodesis versus open reduction and internal fixation for comminuted foot and ankle fractures and treatment of posttraumatic arthritis are also discussed and debated in detail. Last, controversies in the surgical management of the diabetic foot including plastic versus advanced biologics closure and the latest update on the diabetic Charcot foot reconstruction are also reviewed.

The guest editor Dr Blitz and his colleagues were chosen for their surgical expertise and to concisely overview some of the most common controversies and ongoing debates in foot and ankle surgery. I want to thank all the authors, editorial staff, and board members as well as all of the readers for their continuous efforts and support of the *Clinics in Podiatric Medicine and Surgery.*

Thomas Zgonis, DPM
Division of Podiatric Medicine and Surgery
Department of Orthopaedic Surgery
The University of Texas Health Science Center at San Antonio
7703 Floyd Curl Drive–MSC 7776
San Antonio, TX 78229, USA

E-mail address:
zgonis@uthscsa.edu

Clin Podiatr Med Surg 29 (2012) xi
doi:10.1016/j.cpm.2012.04.008
0891-8422/12/$ – see front matter © 2012 Elsevier Inc. All rights reserved.

podiatric.theclinics.com

Preface

Embracing New Technology and Techniques in Foot and Ankle Surgery

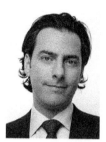

Neal M. Blitz, DPM
Guest Editor

The bulk of our surgical practices involves treating a handful of very common conditions. For the most part, surgeons treat each condition in a rather algorithmic cookie-cutter fashion. There is a tendency to treat most things the same way.

Surgeons may choose "new" procedures that may be considered controversial. But what makes a procedure or technique controversial? New procedures and techniques are often labeled "controversial" because of a lack of follow-up. Interestingly, surgeons adopting new procedures and/or implants are not necessarily considered controversial; rather, they may be seen as contemporary and innovative by patients and their peers.

There are some surgeons who are early adopters of technology and new techniques. Others prefer a "wait-and-see" approach. And there are those surgeons that have their "bags of tricks" and will not modify their practice habits whatsoever.

There is a natural progression for new technology/procedures to become mainstreamed. Change may not be easily accepted, and this sparks controversy and debate. With growing acceptance of new technology, research and medical papers emerge either validating or discrediting the concepts. This *Clinics in Podiatric Medicine and Surgery* highlights several clinical controversies that exist in foot and ankle surgery today.

Neal M. Blitz, DPM
Department of Orthopaedic Surgery
Bronx-Lebanon Hospital Center
Albert Einstein College of Medicine
1650 Grand Concourse, 7th Floor
Bronx, NY 10457, USA

E-mail address:
nealblitz@gmail.com

Clin Podiatr Med Surg 29 (2012) xiii
doi:10.1016/j.cpm.2012.04.007
0891-8422/12/$ – see front matter © 2012 Elsevier Inc. All rights reserved.

podiatric.theclinics.com

End-Stage Hallux Rigidus
Cheilectomy, Implant, or Arthrodesis?

Ruth A. Peace, DPM[a], Graham A. Hamilton, DPM[b],*

KEYWORDS

- Hallux rigidus • Hallux limitus • Arthrodesis • Cheilectomy
- First metatarsophalangeal joint

KEY POINTS

- Hallux rigidus is defined as end-stage arthrosis of the first metatarsophalangeal joint, showing marked limitation of motion and pain with movement and direct pressure.
- The best evidence supports cheilectomy for early-stage arthrosis of the first metatarsophalangeal joint. It cannot, however, be recommended for the treatment of end-stage arthrosis.
- Implants for the great toe joint continue to evolve. Despite good clinical satisfaction, there is still concern about implant survivorship.
- Arthrodesis is the mainstay operative treatment for end-stage hallux rigidus.
- Patients are more likely to return to former activities following arthrodesis compared with implant arthroplasty.

End-stage arthritis of the first metatarsophalangeal joint (MTPJ) typically results in an exophytic process with marked limitation of motion. Pain may occur from the degenerative process itself and/or the bone spur formation that may become directly inflamed from shoe gear. The best surgical treatment for end-stage arthrosis of the big toe joint continues to be a controversial topic despite hallux rigidus being recognized clinically for more than 100 years. Although joint-sparing procedures are considered, joint destructive procedures are recommended, as they are definitive and produce predictable results.

HISTORY OF HALLUX RIGIDUS

Hallux rigidus refers to the limitation of motion at the first MTPJ with particular limitation of hallux dorsiflexion. In 1887, Davies-Colley[1] observed this limitation of motion, calling it *hallux flexus*, because of the relative plantar flexed position of the proximal phalanx in relation to the metatarsal head. Later that same year, Cotterill[2] coined

[a] Kaiser San Francisco Bay Area Foot and Ankle Residency Program, Kaiser Foundation Hospital, 280 West MacArthur Boulevard, Oakland, CA 94611, USA; [b] Department of Orthopedics and Podiatric Surgery, Kaiser Permanente Medical Center, 3400 Delta Fair Boulevard, Antioch, CA 94801, USA
* Corresponding author.
E-mail address: Graham.A.Hamilton@kp.org

Clin Podiatr Med Surg 29 (2012) 341–353
doi:10.1016/j.cpm.2012.04.002
0891-8422/12/$ – see front matter © 2012 Elsevier Inc. All rights reserved.

podiatric.theclinics.com

the term hallux rigidus, still the most commonly used expression for the condition. In 1937, Hiss[3] described the same condition and developed the phrase *hallux limitus*. Although some surgeons consider hallux rigidus and limitus as distinct entities, others consider hallux limitus as an earlier stage of degenerative joint disease, in a continuum of joint degradation.

The painful restricted motion at the first MTPJ is often associated with a mechanical block caused by periarticular osteophytes. The exostosis of the first metatarsal head articulates against an osteophyte at the base of the proximal phalanx leading to mechanical impingement.

ETIOLOGY

The cause of hallux rigidus has not been determined, although multiple predisposing factors have been revealed. Hallux rigidus has been described in 2 different populations: a congenital form and an adult-acquired degenerative form. The congenital form usually presents in the teenage years through the 20s, from a predisposing anatomic factor, such as flattening or squaring of the metatarsal.[4] The adult degenerative form typically presents in a relatively older population in their 40s and 50s, usually as a result of predisposing high-impact activities such as running or dancing. The adult form may be a continuation of the congenital form, although in most cases the exact cause is unknown. The incidence of hallux rigidus in men at age 50 is 31.7% and 40.9% in women of the same age. By age 65, those percentages increase to 51.0% and 67.8%, respectively.[5] Forty-three is shown to be the average age at onset, and the average age at time of surgery is 50 years.[6]

CLASSIFICATION

Numerous investigators have proposed grading systems determined by radiographic changes only, or a combination of clinical and radiographic criteria. Although there are more than 7 classifications used to describe the progressive level of joint arthrosis, none have effectively offered prognostic value, but do offer useful treatment guidelines. The most common clinically used classification system is the Regnauld classification system (**Box 1**).

SURGICAL TREATMENT

Since the original description of hallux rigidus, numerous surgical procedures have been described. Surgical reconstruction for this condition falls into 2 broad categories: those

---

Box 1
Regnauld classification

Grade I: Mild limitation of dorsiflexion, mild dorsal spurring, pain, no sesamoid involvement, subchondral sclerosis, mild sesamoid enlargement

Grade II: Broadening and flattening of the metatarsal head and base of the proximal phalanx, focal joint space narrowing, structural first ray elevatus, osteochondral defect, sesamoid hypertrophy

Grade III: Worsening loss of joint space, near ankylosis, extensive osteophyte formation, osteochondral defects, extensive sesamoid hypertrophy, with or without joint mice

Data from Regnauld B. Disorders of the great toe. In: Elson R, editor. The foot: pathology, etiology, seminology, clinical investigation and treatment. New York: Springer-Verlag; 1986. p. 269–81.

procedures in which the joint is spared and joint-destructive procedures. The latter is typically reserved for joints showing advanced osteoarthritis. Joint-sparing procedures include cheilectomy, phalangeal osteotomy, and first metatarsal osteotomy. Joint-destructive procedures include excisional arthroplasty, implant arthroplasty, and arthrodesis. Newer procedures include a category referred to as cartilage resurfacing: interpositional arthroplasty and arthrodiastasis. The medium-term to long-term efficacy for these procedures by independent researchers has yet to be determined.

Surgery involving the first MTPJ has been present for more than 100 years. Arthrodesis was initially described in 1852 by Broca, but was not popularized for use as treatment for hallux rigidus until 1952 by McKeever.[7] DuVries described the modified cheilectomy,[8] which has remained a popular initial surgical treatment for hallux rigidus. It was not until the 1970s that Swanson popularized the silicone implant.

Although cheilectomy, arthrodesis, and joint replacement are the standards for treatment of this condition, controversy exists as to what stage of hallux rigidus each procedure is best suited. It is well accepted that cheilectomy is indicated in a patient who is in the early stages of clinical symptoms and radiographic joint damage. The joint-destructive procedures are recommended for advanced disease, of which arthrodesis has remained the gold standard.

CHEILECTOMY

Since the original description of hallux rigidus in 1887 by Davies-Colley,[1] variations have existed in the surgical methods of decompressing the MTPJ. It was not until 1959 that DuVries[8] gave a detailed description of the cheilectomy that with modifications is still used by surgeons today. The cheilectomy has become a popular procedure for the treatment of early stages of hallux rigidus in which the major pathology is located at the dorsal aspect of the joint. The procedure is described as the resection of the dorsal 20% to 30% of the metatarsal head.[6,9,10] Joint decompression offers relief of pain while preserving some motion, power, and stability. It also avoids prolonged healing time and it is easily revised, if necessary (**Fig. 1**).[11–13]

The decision as to whether cheilectomy is the appropriate surgical treatment for a specific patient who has hallux rigidus depends on a number of variables. The

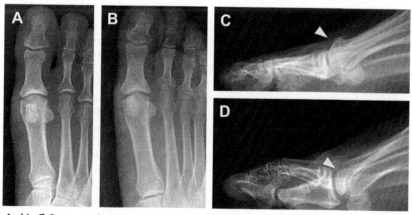

Fig. 1. (*A, C*) Preoperative anteroposterior and lateral radiographs of a 57-year-old woman with mild arthrosis at the first MTPJ. There is no evidence of joint space narrowing (grade I hallux rigidus). (*B, D*) Postoperative anteroposterior and lateral radiographs after resection of the dorsal third of the metatarsal head (*arrow* at metatarsal head).

patient's age, activity level, expectations, and prior treatment history are important, but are not considered as important as the severity of degenerative arthritis. Most of the reports on the surgical outcome of cheilectomy consider hallux rigidus grade as the leading differentiator for recommendation and indication for surgery. Some investigators recommend cheilectomy as a treatment of lower grades only,[6,14–17] whereas others reported successful results even for higher grades of hallux rigidus.[11,12,18] Blitz[14] suggests that cheilectomy is indeed an option for end-stage arthrosis because the dorsal osteophyte is responsible for most pain, and removing this allows for enough pain reduction to satisfy patients' expectations. Nonetheless, cheilectomy is clearly indicated for early stages, grades I and II, using the Regnauld classification scheme.[19,20] Coughlin and Shurnas, however, do not recommend cheilectomy for stages III and IV of their 5-grade classification scheme.[6]

A primary issue associated with cheilectomy is the recurrence of chondrolysis and exostosis as well as further joint deterioration. Easley and colleagues[18] performed 75 cheilectomies using the Hattrup and Johnson classification and American Orthopaedic Foot and Ankle Society (AOFAS) scoring system to evaluate results. The number of patients with grade III increased from 12 to 40 at the 2-year follow-up. Thirty-eight patients worsened at least 1 grade. They also found that the higher the grade at the time of surgery, the less predictable the AOFAS scores became. Patients undergoing cheilectomy should be counseled that given the progressive nature of osteoarthritis, future revisional surgery may be required.

Rates of satisfaction after cheilectomy have been favorable, ranging from 72% and 90%.[11,12,18] Cheilectomy is still a "no bridges burned" type of approach to early-stage hallux rigidus. If the results of cheilectomy prove unsatisfactory, salvage with arthrodesis or resection arthroplasty can be performed in the future.

ARTHROPLASTY

Implant arthroplasty is an alternative surgical option from the standard joint-sparing procedure of a cheilectomy and the joint-destructive procedure of an arthrodesis. The initial attempts and failures at first MTPJ replacement were in the 1950s and did not become widely used until 1965 when Swanson adapted a silicone-stemmed implant. The silicone cap functioned as a spacer following a Keller procedure; this allowed for soft tissue stabilization. In the 1980s, Sutter introduced 2 hinged silastic double-stemmed implants to the market. Sutter's Lawrence and LaPorta gained motion for the mechanical hinge design, whereas the previous Swanson implants gained motion from the viscoelastic properties of the material. These implants temporarily relieved pain, but were not durable. There was mechanical failure of this implant and functionally decreased range of motion. Granberry and colleagues[21] found the frequency of failure to be directly related to the age of the implant. Silicone implants have been associated with many complications, including late failure owing to wear, osteolysis, reactive synovitis, foreign body immune response, and fracture and displacement of components.[22]

Because of the limitations of silicone implants, metallic hemiarthroplasty (unipolar) and metallic total joint arthroplasty (bipolar) prostheses have been developed. Various implants composed of different materials have been manufactured to replace the base of the proximal phalanx, head of the first metatarsal, or both surfaces. Although long-term results of metallic implant hemiarthroplasty have been promising,[23] some investigators continue to consider prosthetic replacement of the first MTPJ as investigational.[24,25]

Some metallic hemiarthroplasty (unipolar) design options for replacement of the base of the proximal phalanx include the Biopro (Biopro Inc, Port Huron, MI), Wright

LPT (Wright Medical technology Inc, Arlington, TN), and Futura (Nexa Orthopedics Inc, San Diego CA) (**Fig. 2**).

A metallic hemiarthroplasty designed for replacement of the head of the first metatarsal, the HemiCAP (Arthrosurface, Franklin, MA), has been available since 2005. The HemiCAP implant is composed of 2 parts: an articular cap made from a cobalt chrome alloy and a central fixation component made of titanium (**Fig. 3**).

Townley and Taranow[23] reported encouraging results with metallic hemiarthroplasty resurfacing for the base of the proximal phalanx using the Biopro implant. A retrospective study of 279 joints resulted in 93.1% excellent (no pain or limitation of activity) results and 2.2% good (occasional discomfort with physical activity) results. Follow-up ranged from 8 months to 33 years. Failures typically occurred within 5 years, and most failures were related to inadequate correction or recurrence of hallux valgus deformity. Failures were also seen in patients with rheumatoid arthritis.

San Giovanni and colleagues[26] reported their preliminary short-term results of first metatarsal head hemiarthroplasty using the HemiCAP (Arthrosurface) implant. Eighty-six patients with 97 implants were reviewed in this multicenter investigation. The mean follow-up was 8 months. The mean AOFAS hallux MTPJ score for 36 cases improved from 49.1 preoperatively to 80.4 postoperatively. Dorsiflexion improved from 26° to 53°.

Metal-on-polyethylene (bipolar) total toe replacement design options have also become available.

Biomet introduced the Koenig total great toe implant in 1988 as a 2-component system that does not require bone cement. Initially a titanium alloy, the newest model is a cobalt-chrome cap with a titanium-sprayed stem that allows for osseointegration into the medullary canal. No independent studies have been performed on this device; however, there is an 83.5% excellent result shown by Koenig and Horwitz.[27] OsteoMed (Addison, TX, USA) created the BioAction Great Toe, which features a metatarsal component constructed of cobalt-chrome, with a phalangeal base component constructed of titanium and polypropylene. Pulavarti and colleagues[28] showed a 77% satisfaction rate with this device. Other implants include the BioPro first MTPJ hemiarthroplasty implant (BioPro), ReFlexion prosthesis (OsteoMed), and Movement Great Toe System (Ascension Orthopedics, Austin, TX, USA).

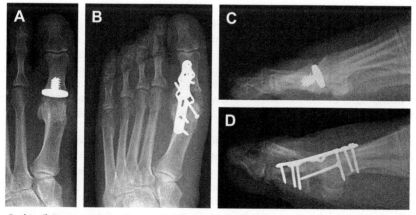

Fig. 2. (*A, C*) Preoperative anteroposterior and lateral radiographs of a 62-year-old woman seen 4 years after a phalangeal hemiarthroplasty. Patient complained of persistent pain and functional limitation in activities of daily living. (*B, D*) The implant was revised with an arthrodesis and ipsilateral calcaneal bone graft.

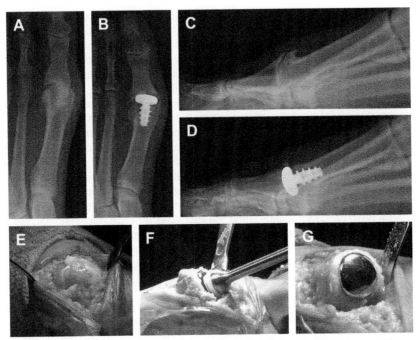

Fig. 3. (A, C) Preoperative anteroposterior and lateral radiographs of a 64-year-old woman with grade III hallux rigidus. The patient underwent a metatarsal head hemiarthroplasty after refusing arthrodesis. (B, D) Postoperative anteroposterior and lateral radiographs at 5 years. There is evidence of bony in-growth slight valgus angulation at the joint and the implant has subsided a few millimeters into the metatarsal head. Despite this suboptimal x-ray, the patient continues to remain very active and walks 2 to 3 miles per day. (E) Intraoperative picture. Note the subtotal loss of hyaline cartilage on the first metatarsal head with exposed subchondral bone. (F, G) Intraoperative picture. The first metatarsal head is debrided of all peripheral osteophytes and reamed for a press fit unipolar implant. The final hemi-implant inserted.

Common complications seen with arthroplasty include pain, osteolysis at the phalanx component, transfer metatarsalgia, foreign body reaction, late failure of the device, and bony overgrowth.[21,28,29] Kim and colleagues[30] showed a 28.3% rate of bony overgrowth (see **Fig. 3**). Loosening of the proximal phalanx component has shown to be a common problem associated with those systems that have a component in the base of the phalanx.[31–33] Owing to the amount of resected bone with arthroplasty, if the system fails, revision arthroplasty or arthrodesis with bone graft are the only reconstruction options.

Unlike the arthrodesis, in which patients are able to return to most of their recreational activities, the total joint replacement has failed to produce similar results. Daniilidis and colleagues[34] showed that there was an overall decrease in recreational sporting activity after the total joint arthroplasty compared with the prearthritic state. This study looked at 23 consecutive patients with grade III hallux rigidus and had 17.4% of patients who were unsatisfied with the outcome at 18 months. The level of dissatisfaction was based on the inability to return to previous recreational activities, secondary to "pain, anxiety, and protection."[34] Patients had the most difficulty returning to high-impact activities like running and soccer.

The first MTPJ replacement systems have improved over the years, but remain investigational. The systems allow retention of motion; however, the results remain unpredictable and the longevity of these joint replacements is not yet known.

ARTHRODESIS

Arthrodesis is considered the benchmark for end-stage osteoarthritis of the first MTPJ.[6] First described for the treatment of hallux valgus in 1894,[35] this procedure has become the standard for advanced hallux rigidus, as it is a "definitive, predictable and viable option."[36] Arthrodesis predictability comes with its reliable union rates, consistent clinical results, and its high rate of patient satisfaction. It is important to counsel the patient that the main goal of the surgical intervention is to provide pain relief, and that arthrodesis will eliminate first MTPJ motion. If the patient and the physician understand this, then the results of surgical intervention can be rewarding. Arthrodesis is best reserved for patients who have an active lifestyle, and after a successful well-positioned fusion, recreational activities that include running can still be expected. However, activities that require hallux en pointe position are mechanically impossible, and shoe wear will be restricted to a heel height less than 2 inches.

Union rates and patient satisfaction have been fairly consistent throughout the literature. Nonunion rates range from 0% to 23%,[37] with current union rates between 91% and 100%.[29] Fixation type has continued to progress over the years with more recent use of plates, locking and nonlocking, that allow for earlier weight bearing. Overall patient satisfaction rates are high.

Coughlin and Shurnas[6] had 100% good or excellent results in 34 patients at 6.7 years. Raikin and colleagues[10] compared arthrodesis and hemiarthroplasty; at 79.4 months, the fusion group had statistically better satisfaction rates. They found that arthrodesis was more reliable in reducing pain and restoring function.

In hallux rigidus, the painful lack of motion at the MTPJ results in lateralization of load-bearing forces during propulsion.[37] Arthrodesis provides consistent results by eliminating painful motion at the joint, as well as providing a stable lever arm for propulsion. Brodsky and colleagues[38] followed 23 patients prospectively after first MTPJ arthrodesis. At 1 year, there was a statistically significant increase in maximal ankle push-off power and single-limb support time, and a decrease in step width, showing an "improvement in propulsive power, weight-bearing function of the foot, and stability during gait."

Stability provided to the foot and the elimination of painful motion allows individuals to return to most of their recreational sporting activities. In their 1996 case study, Bouche and Adad[36] showed that first MTPJ arthrodesis in active patients could "relieve pain and allow patients to perform some athletic function (including running)." All 5 of the individuals, age range from 42 to 57 years, were able to return to their respective preoperative activities, which included walking, exercise, race walking, power walking, and running. Mann[39] noted minimal effect on a patient's gait after arthrodesis and is evident in patient return to activity.

Although a joint-destructive procedure, arthrodesis is "a successful surgical procedure that provides relief of pain, correction of deformity and allows a high level of function in everyday life and in recreational activities."[40]

Authors' Recommended Procedure and Surgical Technique

The most compelling argument for first MTPJ arthrodesis versus implant arthroplasty for end-stage hallux rigidus, comes from a head-to-head comparison of these 2 surgical options conducted by Gibson and Thompson.[33] In a randomized control trial, first MTPJ arthrodesis had a significantly greater improvement of symptoms at 2 years compared with those who underwent arthroplasty with a Biomet unconstrained total joint. Twenty-two patients (38 toes) had arthrodesis and 27 patients (39 toes) had arthroplasty. Thirteen of the arthroplasty patients had continued problems with swelling at 6 months. Six of those 13 underwent revisional surgery. At 18 months into the trial, 5 of the 30 patients having undergone arthroplasty were having significant joint pain, with radiolucency noted around the component in the base of the proximal phalanx, indicating loosening of the component. Two were revised at this point and the remaining implants were placed using bone cement. In the arthrodesis group, 2 patients felt that they were aware of walking on the outsides of their feet; 9 were prescribed rocker-bottom–soled shoes. Based on this study, it is the authors' recommendation to treat end-stage hallux rigidus with an arthrodesis procedure.

Authors' Preferred Surgical Technique for Arthrodesis

A standard curvilinear incision is made medial to the long extensor tendon. It should extend from just proximal to the hallux interphalangeal joint crossing the MTPJ and extend proximally to about midshaft on the first metatarsal (**Fig. 4**). The entire incision is usually 8 to 9 cm in length. The more extensile incision allows for easier application of the implants, in particular the plate. If previous scars are present, then an attempt should be made to make the incision along these previous scar lines. The joint is

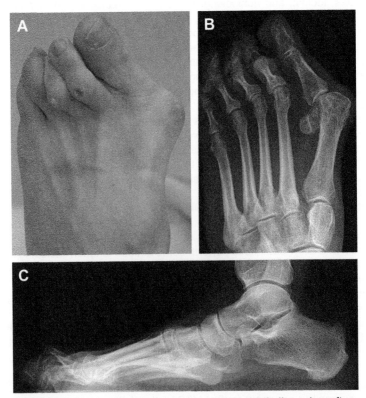

Fig. 4. (A) Clinical picture of a 67-year-old woman with severe hallux valgus, first ray hypermobility, and lesser digital clawtoe deformities. Patient could not tolerate a non–weight-bearing convalescence. (B, C) Anteroposterior and lateral radiographs of the patient's foot.

entered through a dorsal arthrotomy and the head of the first metatarsal and base of the proximal phalanx is exposed. With severely subluxed or dislocated sesamoids, a release of the conjoint adductor tendon is also required in the first interspace. The authors prefer using a conical reaming system for joint preparation. Once all the dorsal osteophytes are removed, a guide pin is then placed in the center of the first metatarsal head and base of the proximal phalanx; the ball and socket reamers are used to remove all joint cartilage and subchondral bone (**Fig. 5**). It is important to ream without using power instrumentation, so as to avoid overzealous removal of bone, particularly in the rheumatoid patient or patient with a poorer bone stock. Attaching the reamer to a chuck handle and controlled clockwise rotation affords excellent joint preparation. Using this technique allows for rapid joint preparation, and provides a large bone surface area for fusion. It also affords an excellent ball-and-socket fit with little to no gapping.

With the joint prepared, functional positioning is then required. The authors have found in cases where a large intermetatarsal (IM) angle is present, a percutaneous 2.0-mm wire can first be inserted to translate the first metatarsal laterally and reduce the IM angle.

The functional position of the hallux is then assessed by loading the entire foot on a flat surface (tray cover). The toe is placed in slight dorsiflexion (contacting the load-bearing surface), slight valgus (parallel with the second toe) and with no frontal plane rotation (nail should be straight up). This position is desired to simulate a functional "toe-off" position, once fusion has been attained. With the toe positioned correctly, it is temporarily stabilized with a 2.0-mm Kirschner-wire. The position can be checked intraoperatively using fluoroscopy or C-arm. In the anteroposterior view, the IM angle should be reduced; the sesamoids should be relocated under the first metatarsal. A congruent fit should be present at the first MTPJ with the hallux parallel with the second digit (approximately 10–15° of valgus). On the lateral projection, the hallux should be approximately 30° to the long axis of the first metatarsal, or 10° to 15° to the load-bearing surface.

In some cases, positioning can be challenging, such as in cases with a cross-over second toe deformity or hallux valgus interphalangeus. In the case of the cross-over second toe deformity, this should be addressed first and, once relocated, pinned across the lesser second MTPJ so as to better assess hallux position in the transverse plane. In the case of the hallux interphalangeus, clinical position overrides radiographic position. Clinically, the hallux is positioned parallel to the second digit.

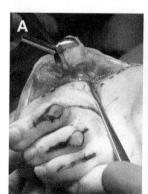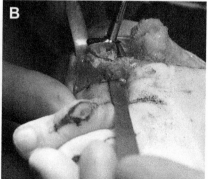

Fig. 5. (*A, B*) Clinical pictures of joint preparation using conical reamers. Note reaming is done by hand to avoid overzealous bone loss.

Radiographically, this usually demonstrates on the anteroposterior view as a first MTPJ that is rectus (straight) or in slight varus. For these cases, such a position is optimal for fusion, as opposed to in slight valgus. If a slight valgus position is obtained, patients will complain of lateral hallux impingement with the second toe and callus formation.

Once the corrected functional position has been obtained, and confirmed on intraoperative imaging, definitive fixation is performed (**Fig. 6**). First, a cortical lag screw is placed. Here screw diameters are either 3.5-mm or 4.0-mm solid screws and usually run 28 mm to 40 mm in length. Many options are available as far as screw direction. It can be inserted either from the medial aspect of the first metatarsal or from the medial base of the proximal phalanx. Cannulated screws can also be used. Screw direction from the first metatarsal to the hallux is the preferred option, as this will cause interfragmentary compression of the fusion site with a slight valgus thrust. Directing the screw from the medial aspect of the hallux to the lateral metatarsal can cause the toe to shift into a slight varus alignment as the screw is tightened. With the lag screw placed, a dorsal neutralization plate is then contoured to the dorsal surface of the first metatarsal and proximal phalanx. A standard one-third tubular plate can be used, ensuring at least 4 cortices are engaged with compression screws proximal and distal to the joint line.

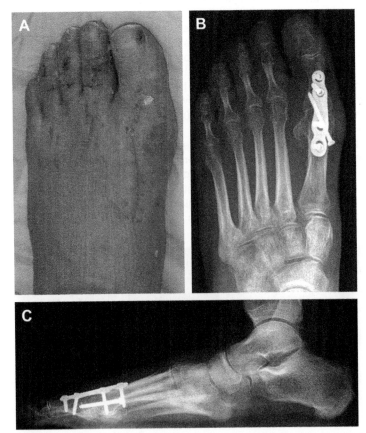

Fig. 6. (*A*) Clinical weight-bearing image of patient at 6 weeks. (*B*, *C*) Anteroposterior and lateral weight-bearing radiographs at 6 weeks.

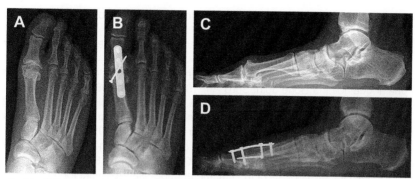

Fig. 7. (*A, C*) Preoperative radiographs of a 52-year-old man with grade III hallux rigidus. (*B, D*) Postoperative radiographs with solid union at 8 weeks after fusion with a single lag screw and dorsal plate.

In the patient with more porotic bone, a locking fixed-angle plate can be used. There are also many commercially available low-profile precontoured fixed angle specialty plates. These certainly can be beneficial in the patient with poorer bone stock, but they are not required in all cases (**Fig. 7**).

Postoperatively

With the advent of newer implants, patients have the ability to ambulate on the foot almost immediately after surgery. Our protocol is a fracture shoe or walking boot for 6 weeks. The offloading device is decided on based on the stability of the arthrodesis construct and the integrity of the bone stock. This protocol is consistent with other investigators. Dayton and McCall[41] walked all of their 18 patients immediately after fusion in a postoperative shoe. Union was achieved on average in 6.1 weeks and patients were on average in an athletic shoe at 6.23 weeks. Hyer and colleagues[42] reported similar findings; 37 patients were allowed to bear weight immediately, with a fusion rate of 91.1%.

SUMMARY

Although controversy still exists in procedure selection in cases of moderate arthrosis of the first MTPJ, there is consensus that in cases of early joint destruction, cheilectomy affords favorable results. The literature shows variance on duration of symptomatic relief after cheilectomy, but across the board, there is pain relief, increased range of motion, and there is no limitation in future surgical revision options.

With end-stage hallux rigidus, the biomedical literature advocates arthrodesis over cheilectomy and implant arthroplasty. Biomechanically, first MTPJ arthrodesis causes little to no disability with transfer stresses to the remaining joints and has little adverse effect on gait. Arthrodesis restores the weight-bearing function of the first ray with increased force carried through the hallux at toe-off. Regardless of classification system used, the results after first MTPJ arthrodesis are consistent and predictable with high patient satisfaction.

REFERENCES

1. Davies-Colley N. Contraction of the metatarsophalangeal joint of the great toe. Br Med J 1887;1:728.

2. Cotterill JM. Condition of stiff great toe in adolescents. Edinburgh Med J 1887;33: 459–62.
3. Hiss JM. Functional foot disorders. Los Angeles: Los Angeles Press Company; 1937. p. 251–9.
4. Sheriff MJ, Baumhauer JF. Hallux rigidus and osteoarthrosis of the first metatarsophalangeal joint. J Bone Joint Surg Am 1998;80(6):898–908.
5. Van Saase JL, Van Romunde LK, Cats A, et al. Epidemiology of osteoarthritis: Zoetermeer survey. Comparison of radiological osteoarthritis in a Dutch population with that in 10 other populations. Ann Rheum Dis 1989;48:271–80.
6. Coughlin MJ, Shurnas PS. Hallux rigidus: grading and long-term results of operative treatment. J Bone Joint Surg Am 2003;85(11):2072–88.
7. McKeever DC. Arthrodesis of the first metatarsophalangeal joint for hallux valgus, hallux rigidus, and metatarsus primus varus. J Bone Joint Surg Am 1952;34: 129–34.
8. DuVries H. Static deformities. DuVries' Surgery of the foot. St Louis (MO): Mosby; 1959. p. 392–8.
9. Beeson P. The surgical treatment of hallux limitus/rigidus: a critical review of the literature. Foot 2004;14:6–22.
10. Raikin SM, Ahmad J, Pour AE, et al. Comparison of arthrodesis and metallic hemiarthroplasty of the hallux metatarsophalangeal joint. J Bone Joint Surg Am 2007; 89(9):1979–85.
11. Mann RA, Coughlin MJ, Duvries HL. Hallux rigidus: a review of the literature and a method of treatment. Clin Orthop 1979;142:57–63.
12. Mann RA, Clanton TO. Hallux rigidus: treatment by surgical cheilectomy. J Bone Joint Surg 1988;70A(3):400–6.
13. Roukis TS. Review article: the need for surgical revision after isolated cheilectomy for hallux rigidus: a systematic review. J Foot Ankle Surg 2010;49:465–70.
14. Blitz N. Is cheilectomy an option for end-stage hallux rigidus? Podiatry Today. Available at: http://www.podiatrytoday.com/blogged/is-cheilectomy-an-option-for-end-stage-hallux-rigidus. Accessed February 10, 2012.
15. Smith RW, Katchis SD, Ayson LC. Outcomes in hallux rigidus patients treated non-operatively: a long-term follow-up study. Foot Ankle Int 2000;21(11):906–13.
16. Gould N. Hallux rigidus: cheilectomy of implant. Foot Ankle Int 1981;315–20.
17. Feldman RS, Hutter J, Lapow L, et al. Cheilectomy and hallux rigidus. J Foot Ankle Surg 1983;22:170–4.
18. Easley ME, Davis WH, Anderson RB. Intermediate to long-term follow-up of medial-approach dorsal cheilectomy for hallux rigidus. Foot Ankle Int 1999;20:147–52.
19. Waizy H, Abbara-Czardybon M, Stukenborg-Colsman C, et al. Mid- and long-term results of the joint preserving therapy of hallux rigidus. Arch Orthop Trauma Surg 2010;130(2):165–70.
20. Yee G, Lau J. Current concepts review: hallux rigidus. Foot Ankle Int 2008;6: 637–46.
21. Granberry WM, Noble PC, Bishop JO, et al. Use of a hinged silicone prosthesis for replacement arthroplasty of the first metatarsophalangeal joint. J Bone Joint Surg Am 1991;73(10):1453–9.
22. Esway JE, Conti SF. Joint replacement in the hallux MTPJ. Foot Ankle Clin 2005; 10:97–115.
23. Townley CO, Taranow WS. A metallic hemiarthroplasty resurfacing prosthesis for the hallux MTPJ. Foot Ankle Int 1994;15:575–80.
24. Brage ME, Ball ST. urgical options for salvage of end-stage hallux rigidus. Foot Ankle Clin 2002;7:49–73.

25. Keiserman LS, Sammarco VJ. Surgical treatment of the hallux rigidus. Foot Ankle Clin 2005;10:75–96.
26. San Giovanni TP, Graf U, Shields N, et al. Pain relief and function improvement with metatarsal resurfacing in hallux rigidus: preliminary results in a multicenter case series with a surgical alternative to fusion. Arthrosurface 2007.
27. Koenig RD, Horwitz LR. The Biomet Total Toe System utilizing the Koenig score: a five-year review. J Foot Ankle Surg 1996;35(1):23–6.
28. Pulavarti RS, McVie JL, Tulloch CJ. First metatarsophalangeal joint replacement using the bio-action great toe implant: intermediate results. Foot Ankle Int 2005;26(12):1033–7.
29. DeCarbo WT, Lupica J, Hyer CF. Modern techniques in hallux rigidus surgery. Clin Podiatr Med Surg 2011;28:361–83.
30. Kim PJ, Hatch D, DiDomenico LA, et al. A multicenter retrospective review of outcomes for arthrodesis, hemi-metallic joint implant, and resectional arthroplasty in the surgical treatment of end-stage hallux rigidus. J Foot Ankle Surg 2012; 51(1):50–60.
31. Swanson AB. Implant arthroplasty for the great toe. Clin Orthop Relat Res 1972; 85:75–81.
32. Fuhrmann RA, Wagner A, Anders JO. First metatarsophalangeal joint replacement: the method of choice for end stage hallux rigidus? Foot Ankle Clin 2003; 8:711–21.
33. Gibson JN, Thompson CE. Arthrodesis or total replacement arthroplasty for hallux rigidus: a randomized control trial. Foot Ankle Int 2005;26(9):680–90.
34. Daniilidis K, Martinelli N, Marinozzi A, et al. Recreational sporting activity after total replacement of the first metatarsophalangeal joint: a prospective study. Int Orthop 2010;34:973–9.
35. Clutton HH. The treatment of hallux valgus. St Thomas Rep 1894;22:1–12.
36. Bouche RT, Adad JM. Arthrodesis of the first metatarsophalangeal joint in active people. Clin Podiatr Med Surg 1996;13:461–84.
37. Hamilton G, Ford L, Patel S. First metatarsophalangeal joint arthrodesis and revision arthrodesis. Clin Podiatr Med Surg 2009;26:459–73.
38. Brodsky J, Baum B, Pollo F, et al. Prospective gait analysis in patients with first metatarsophalangeal joint arthrodesis for hallux rigidus. Foot Ankle Int 2007; 28(2):162–5.
39. Mann RA. Surgical implications of biomechanics of the foot and ankle. Clinc Orthop Relat Res 1980;146:111–8.
40. Brodsky JW, Passmore RN, Pollo FE, et al. Functional outcome of arthrodesis of the first metatarsophalangeal joint using parallel screw fixation. Foot Ankle Int 2005;26:140–6.
41. Dayton P, McCall A. Early weightbearing after first metatarsophalangeal joint arthrodesis: a retrospective observational case analysis. J Foot Ankle Surg 2004;43(3):156–9.
42. Hyer CF, Berlet GB, Glover JP. A retrospective review of immediate weightbearing after first metatarsophalangeal joint arthrodesis. Foot Ankle Spec 2008;1(1):24–8.

Hammertoe Surgery
Arthroplasty, Arthrodesis or Plantar Plate Repair?

Klaus J. Kernbach, DPM

KEYWORDS

- Hammertoe deformity • Conservative care • Surgical management

KEY POINTS

- A thorough history and physical examination of the lower extremity is paramount to an appropriate diagnosis and evaluation of the cause of hammertoe and best treatment course.
- Hammertoe deformity is a common problem that responds well to conservative care in most cases. If conservative care fails, then surgery may be considered in the absence of peripheral arterial disease.
- Concomitant structural anatomic problems (metatarsus primus varus, hallux abductovalgus, first ray hypermobility, equinus, plantar plate attenuation, and degenerative joint disease) should be readily diagnosed and managed as symptomatic hammertoe deformity may be exacerbated by these conditions.

Hammertoe deformity is defined as dorsiflexion of the proximal phalanx on the metatarsal head at the metatarsal phalangeal joint (MTPJ), and plantarflexion of the intermediate phalanx on the proximal phalanx at the proximal interphalangeal joint (PIPJ).[1] The distal interphalangeal joint (DIPJ) may be dorsiflexed, plantarflexed, or in a neutral position (**Fig. 1**).[2] Contracture of the involved joints can be rigid, semirigid, or flexible. In severe instances of hammertoe deformity, dislocation or subluxation of the MTPJ can occur and this can further exacerbate the condition by placing retrograde pressure onto the plantar MTPJ, thereby causing further attenuation of the plantar plate with a distal migration of the plantar fat pad in a vicious circle (**Fig. 2**).

Painful hammertoe deformity and lesser MTPJ pain are commonplace in a foot specialist's clinical practice. These complaints are frequently interrelated and exist concomitantly with first ray hypermobility, metarsus primus elevatus, metatarsus primus varus, metatarsal parabola abnormalities (with a negative first metatarsal protrusion distance), hallux abductovalus, gastrocnemius equinus, and obesity-driven forefoot overload syndrome.[3] Hyperkeratotic lesions are often present on the dorsal apex of the hammertoe deformity, distal toe tip, and/or at the plantar MTPJ. Onychodystrophy may develop due to repetitive micro-trauma on the nail matrix secondary to the hammertoe contracture deformity. A modified Lachman test, also called a dorsal drawer

Kaiser North Bay Consortium Residency Program, Department of Podiatry, Kaiser Foundation Hospital, 975 Sereno Drive, Vallejo, CA 94589, USA
E-mail address: kkernbach@gmail.com

Clin Podiatr Med Surg 29 (2012) 355–366
doi:10.1016/j.cpm.2012.04.006
0891-8422/12/$ – see front matter © 2012 Elsevier Inc. All rights reserved.

podiatric.theclinics.com

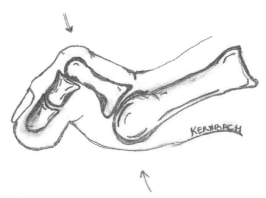

Fig. 1. Hammertoe deformity with arrows depicting the dorsal and plantar apices of deformity that can be overloaded from shoe gear pressure and ground reactive force. Plantar plate attenuation and a distal migration of the plantar fat pad are not uncommon in these circumstances.

test, should be used to evaluate for the presence of MTPJ predislocation syndrome.[4] A comprehensive physical examination should also include an evaluation of all painful regions, hammertoe flexibility, first ray hypermobility, the Silfverskiold test for gastrocnemius equinus, and any open and closed kinetic chain differences in the reduction of deformity.[3,5,6] Special care should be taken to differentiate the diagnosis of neuroma from the more common diagnosis of mechanically-induced MTPJ predislocation syndrome.

Trauma, neuromuscular disorders, and inflammatory arthropathies such as rheumatoid or psoriatic arthritis can further exacerbate the hammertoe condition. These etiologies should be considered in the workup with a comprehensive history, review of systems, physical examination, and imaging. Diagnostic imaging should include weight-bearing dorsoplantar, plantar-axial, and lateral plain film radiographs, which may elucidate early lesser MTPJ subluxation/dislocation and first ray insufficiency. Arthrography of the symptomatic MTPJ and/or magnetic resonance imaging (MRI)

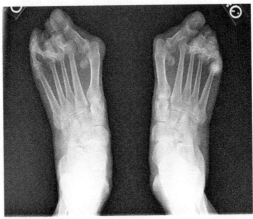

Fig. 2. Weight-bearing dorsoplantar radiograph of chronic lesser MTPJ dislocations and hammertoes associated with inadequately corrected metatarsus primus varus, hallux valgus, and long central metatarsals. Gastrocnemius equinus was also present clinically.

should be considered in cases where acute plantar plate rupture or attenuation is suspected.[5,7] Blitz and colleagues[7] identified anatomic variances in second MTPJ arthrography and suggested that arthrography be performed under fluoroscopic guidance and correlated with the clinical scenario. If the contralateral foot is asymptomatic, consideration should be given for its use as an arthrography comparison control with an identical injection technique.

If there is a lack of digital hair and/or decreased peripheral pulses, then noninvasive vascular studies should be considered as part of the hammertoe workup. Doppler ultrasonography with toe-brachial index (TBI) and/or transcutaneous oxygen pressure measurement can be used to elucidate peripheral arterial disease (PAD) in the distal forefoot. If PAD is present, a complete evaluation with an appropriate vascular specialist should be completed before any invasive hammertoe procedure is considered.

Conservative care for chronic hammertoe deformity with associated lesser MTPJ pain includes padding, arch supports with associated top cover modifications, a rigid rocker-soled extra-depth shoe or walking boot, nonsteroidal antiinflammatory drugs, and weight loss when indicated. Padding options may include crest-buttress pads, tube foam, lamb's wool, and/or silicon gel pads. Strict avoidance of barefoot walking, especially on hard surfaces, and placement of rugs in high traffic areas where barefoot walking or standing occurs can also help to improve the symptoms of lesser MTPJ pain. A Budin splint or Gerard Yu figure-of-eight toe strapping can also be effective in ameliorating symptoms (**Fig. 3**).[4] In contrast to the Budin splint, toe strapping with tape has a lower profile, which allows for its use with arch supports and accompanying cushioned top covers. Intra-articular lesser MTPJ cortisone injection may actually propagate an acute-on-chronic plantar plate rupture[5] and should be used judiciously under limited circumstances with protected weight bearing and concurrent toe strapping (see **Fig. 3**) for a minimum of 6 weeks.

When conservative treatment fails, surgical options for hammertoe correction can be divided into resectional arthroplasty, arthrodesis, or plantar plate repair. Hammertoes and lesser MTPJ pain may occur in isolation, or may be secondary to first ray insufficiency (ie, hallux valgus deformity). When hallux valgus is present, it must also be treated concurrently to adequately correct the position of the second toe and

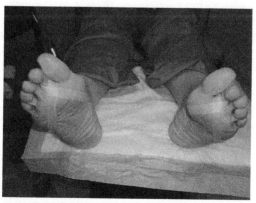

Fig. 3. Bilateral Gerard Yu figure-of-eight toe strapping with 12-mm (0.5-in) paper tape placed on the base of the second toes to reduce hyperextension deformity at the MTPJ.[4] Similar strapping can also be applied to the third toes as needed. This strapping is easy to perform and can be both diagnostic and therapeutic in its efficacy for treatment of predislocation syndrome.

prevent recurrence.[2,3,8] In cases of complex hammertoe deformity with lesser MTPJ pain, consideration should also be given to central metatarsal decompressional shortening osteotomies.[2–4] Further consideration should be given to gastrocnemius recession when pathologic gastrocnemius equinus is present and contributing to increased forefoot load and thereby, lesser MTPJ pain and deformity.[3,5]

ARTHROPLASTY

Hammertoe repair by means of simple proximal phalangeal head resection without Kirschner wire (K-wire) transfixation may lead to digital instability and/or malalignment secondary to tendon imbalance,[2] particularly in the second and third toe. Isolated PIPJ resectional arthroplasty does not address the sagittal plane deformity that typically exists concomitantly at the MTPJ. This has led some surgeons to advocate for single-stage MTPJ capsular tendinous rebalancing, plantar plate repair,[5,9,10] PIPJ resectional arthroplasty and/or fusion with K-wire transfixation across the MTPJ.[2,11,12] In cases of hammertoe deformity with incongruity at the MTPJ, consideration should be given for open reduction of the MTPJ deformity with K-wire splintage and/or metatarsal shortening osteotomies when indicated.[2,8,12]

O'Kane and Kilmartin[8] retrospectively reviewed 75 patients (100 toes) with an average age of 63 years who had an excisional second toe PIPJ arthroplasty without K-wire transfixation or MTPJ joint capsule release at an average of 44 months follow-up. They reported mean preoperative and postoperative AOFAS (American Orthopaedic Foot and Ankle Society) scoring of 46 and 94, respectively. However, 53 feet had adjunctive hallux valgus repair and 16 feet required both hallux valgus repair and a second metatarsal osteotomy. There were also 35 excisional arthroplasties on adjacent toes. Hence, the results of their scoring analysis were biased by the ancillary surgical procedures and not the isolated second toe PIPJ arthroplasty alone. The investigators cite the rapid return to some variety of footwear and activity at 2 weeks postoperatively as advantages to performing this PIPJ resectional arthroplasty without pinning. They further identify that the digit maintains some degree of desirable flexion after arthroplasty as another advantage. However, 31% of the toes in their study had various complications with floating toe the most common.[8]

Arthroplasty with K-wire splintage maintained for 6 weeks commonly results in a clinical outcome similar to PIPJ arthrodesis (**Figs. 4–8**). Coughlin and colleagues,[11] in their review of 118 PIPJ resectional arthroplasties performed with intramedullary K-wire transfixation, found that 81% of the toes went onto PIPJ fusion and the remaining 19% had a fibrous union. In the absence of pain and instability, a fibrous union is not an indication for revisional surgery.[2,11]

Arthroplasty without K-wire splintage for hammertoe deformity can sometimes be effective. In circumstances of fourth or fifth hammertoe deformity with adductovarus rotation, simple PIPJ resectional arthroplasty without pinning is frequently beneficial in ameliorating symptomatic hyperkeratotic lesions (**Figs. 9 and 10**).

ARTHRODESIS

In cases of symptomatic rigid hammertoe deformity, proximal interphalangeal joint arthrodesis (PIPJA) has been the mainstay of corrective surgery.[13–16] It has been reported that PIPJA provides better toe purchase with increased stability and sagittal plane correction than simple PIPJ resectional arthroplasty without K-wire transfixation.[16] End-to-end PIPJA is the most common procedure for hammertoe correction.[13,14] Peg-in-hole PIPJ fusion has also been used.[16–18] Miller and colleagues[15] have advocated a chevron modification to the end-to-end PIPJA, citing the increased

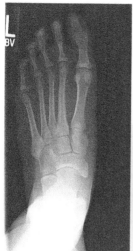
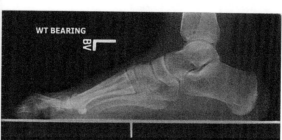

Fig. 4. Weight-bearing preoperative dorsoplantar and lateral radiographs. Note the hammering of digits 2 to 5 with long second and third metatarsals. The patient's toes were symptomatic with a positive dorsal drawer test and painful exuberant hyperkeratotic lesions at the plantar second and third MTPJ. A gastrocnemius equinus was also present clinically.

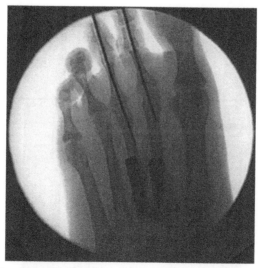

Fig. 5. Intraoperative fluoroscopic image. The following procedures were performed: (1) gastrocnemius intra-aponeurotic recession; (2) second and third metatarsal cylindrical decompressional shortening osteotomies; (3) PIPJ arthroplasty of the second toe with K-wire transfixation across the MTPJ; (4) DIPJ arthroplasty of the third toe with K-wire transfixation across the MTPJ; (5) stab flexor tenotomies of the fourth and fifth toes (not yet performed at the time of this fluoroscopic image). With plantarflexion of the second and third toes at the MTPJ, the joint spaces appear narrowed secondary to parallax. The patient's contralateral right lower extremity had nearly identical deformities that were corrected 7 months earlier with similar procedures that she was satisfied with.

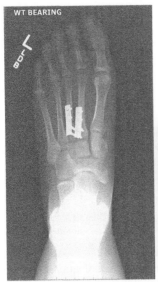

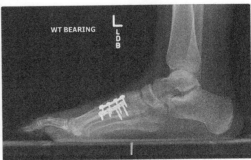

Fig. 6. Weight-bearing postoperative dorsoplantar and lateral radiographs. The K-wires were removed on postoperative day 38. An asymptomatic fibrous union was present at the second and third toe interphalangeal joints. The patient's plantar second and third MTPJ pain and callus resolved with an improvement in the metatarsal parabola, hammertoe, and equinus deformity.

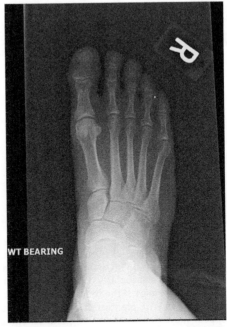

Fig. 7. Weight-bearing preoperative dorsoplantar radiograph with a lesion marker representing the symptomatic hyperkeratotic fourth interdigital space lesion.

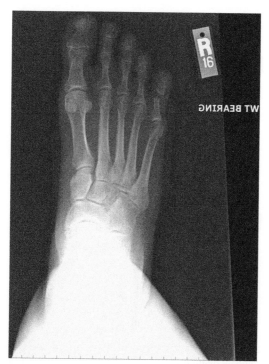

Fig. 8. Weight-bearing postoperative dorsoplantar radiograph after resectional derotational arthroplasty of the fifth toe PIPJ without pinning. This procedure ameliorated the painful interdigital lesion.

cancellous bone surface area contact and increased construct stability as two surgical benefits. Disadvantages of their technique, in comparison to end-to-end PIPJA technique, include the need for more exposure at the base of the intermediate phalanx to make the bone cuts, and additional bone resection which further shortens the toe.[15]

A multitude of fixation methods for PIPJA have been described including standard percutaneous K-wire,[2,11] buried K-wire,[19] threaded K-wire,[15] absorbable fixation rod,[15,20] catgut suture,[21] 20-guage stainless steel wire suture,[22] and screw fixation.[23] Traditional K-wire splintage is still the easiest, most efficient and most cost-effective method for hammertoe correction in this author's opinion. Absorbable fixation can be considered when the patient has a metal allergy.[20]

Mallet toe and hyperextension of the PIPJ have been identified as potential complications after a PIPJ fusion.[11,12,24] It has been reported that the use of intramedullary K-wire transfixation for periods greater than 3 weeks may lead to increased rates of infection and wire breakage.[25] Use of 1.6-mm (0.062-in) K-wires, rather than 1.1-mm (0.045-in) K-wires, helps to prevent unwanted breakage, which is more common with the thinner diameter K-wires during weight bearing cyclical loading moments. In pediatric hammertoe correction, or with very petite patients, use of 1.1-mm K-wires may be considered.

Depending on the ancillary procedures performed, use of a short-leg walking cast with a long toe box, versus an oversized postoperative shoe, helps to protect the K-wire and prevent unwanted wire migration. To help prevent K-wire migration and sharps injury, the K-wire should be bent, cut transversely (as opposed to obliquely)

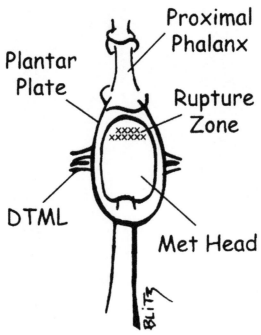

Fig. 9. The rupture zone of the plantar plate. DTML, deep transverse intermetatarsal ligament; Met Head, metatarsal head. (*Modified from* Blitz NM, Ford LA, Christensen JC. Plantar plate repair of the second metatarsophalangeal joint: technique and tips. J Foot Ankle Surg 2004;43:266–70; with permission.)

and then capped. In all cases of hammertoe repair, careful postoperative monitoring of the digit should be performed. In some cases, removal of the K-wire may be required to prevent vascular embarrassment with overzealous reduction.

PLANTAR PLATE REPAIR

The plantar plate is an important restraint that resists MTPJ subluxation/dislocation.[26,27] Commonly, MTPJ plantar plate pathology is associated with hammertoe deformity and this has led to some controversy regarding the best treatment strategy. Ford and colleagues[9] identified plantar plate repair (PPR) as a specific approach to treat hammertoes that are unstable in the sagittal plane at the level of the MTPJ. Blitz and colleagues[10] further elucidated a specific surgical technique for PPR.

Although hammertoe correction with PPR has been advocated, few studies on PPR exist.[5,9,28,29] In one of the largest series on plantar plate repair to date, Bouche and Heit[5] performed open PPR and hammer toe correction with flexor digitorum longus tendon transfer (FDLT) in 18 patients (20 feet) with chronic sagittal plane instability of the lesser MTPJ. In all cases, a plantar longitudinal incision was made to expose the plantar plate. PPR were performed with a 3-0 absorbable suture on a tapered needle in an end-to-end technique for tears in the midsubstance region. If the plantar plate tear was present at the distal insertion on the proximal phalangeal base then a minianchor was used for PPR. Ancillary procedures were performed. In all cases, PIPJ arthrodesis or arthroplasty were performed with K-wire transfixation for 6 weeks. Distal metaphyseal metatarsal osteotomy was also performed when indicated. All patients were typically non–weight bearing on crutches for up to 6 weeks, depending on the

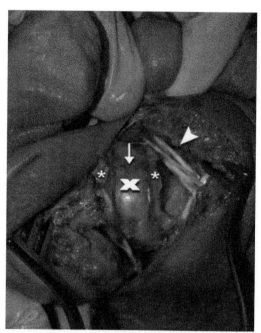

Fig. 10. Cadaveric specimen of the intact plantar plate. The rupture zone (X) is located just proximal to insertion of the plantar plate onto the base of the proximal phalanx (*arrow*). The incised flexor sheath (*asterisks*) is continuous with the plantar plate. The flexor tendons (*arrowhead*) are retracted laterally. (*Modified from* Blitz NM, Ford LA, Christensen JC. Plantar plate repair of the second metatarsophalangeal joint: technique and tips. J Foot Ankle Surg 2004;43:266–70; with permission.)

procedures performed. The average postoperative AOFAS score was 83.2 (range 57–100) and the average postoperative follow-up was 36.9 months (range 12–66 months).[5]

Lui and colleagues,[28] from Hong Kong, reported on a modified plantar plate tenodesis for correction of claw toe deformity. They initially performed the modified plantar plate tenodesis in 10 fresh cadaveric feet by anchoring the plantar plate of the second MTPJ to the extensor digitorum longus (EDL) tendon by utilizing figure-of-eight suture. This plantar plate tenodesis technique was complicated by tethering of the flexor tendon sheath in 2 specimens. In the clinical study of 23 patients, 2 separate operative techniques were compared. They used MTPJ arthroscopy to evaluate plantar plate integrity. Avascular necrosis of the second metatarsal head developed after their modified plantar plate tenodesis and the technique was subsequently re-modified after the complication occurred. Flexor tendon tethering may still have occurred in the clinical group as well.[28]

Ford and colleagues[9] performed a cadaveric comparison of PPR and flexor digitorum longus (FDL) tendon transfer procedures in cases of digital instability. Although they identified that both PPR and FDL tendon transfer procedures were effective, they surmised that a combination of both procedures would be most effective for stabilizing the MTPJ. This was consistent with the findings of Bouche and Heit[5] who confided that their results with isolated FDL tendon transfer or PPR alone were suboptimal. Isolated acute or subacute plantar plate tears may be treated with primary repair without concomitant procedures. After PPR, the patient should be prepared for a longer period of forefoot offloading than would be expected with PIPJA alone.

SUMMARY

In cases of painful complex hammertoe deformity, there is no single approach that can be used in all circumstances. If conservative care fails, surgical management may include arthroplasty, arthrodesis, and/or plantar plate repair. The best and most pragmatic surgical plan must be patient-centered, taking the age, activity level, and expectations of the patient into account.

In the geriatric patient with low functional demands, simple arthroplasty or elective hammertoe amputation can ameliorate symptoms with a faster recovery while decreasing the potential for catastrophic fall risk complications. Simple derotational PIPJ arthroplasty can also be effective in treating symptomatic hyperkeratotic lesions on the fourth and fifth toes. A preoperative lesion marker should be used to further scrutinize the precise cause of symptomatic lesions, particularly those in the interdigital spaces.

In cases of chronic neuropathic ulceration secondary to hammertoe deformity, simple resectional arthroplasty can be considered without K-wire transfixation. If percutaneous stab flexor tenotomy fails, or in cases of rigid PIPJ contracture where flexor tenotomy with closed reduction would not be effective, resectional arthroplasty can be beneficial. Whenever possible, digital neuropathic ulceration secondary to hammertoe deformity should be healed with appropriate offloading before surgical hammertoe correction is performed. Appropriate noninvasive vascular evaluation with a TBI should be performed when indicated. In cases involving complex medical conditions, crossover toe deformity with dislocation, and/or chronic digital ulceration, consideration should be given to primary amputation of the affected digit in lieu of hammertoe reconstruction.

In an active patient with symptomatic rigid second or third digital hammertoe deformity, interphalangeal joint arthrodesis or arthroplasty with K-wire transfixation for 4 to 6 weeks can reliably improve symptoms. There is increasing evidence that concomitant PPR can also be considered when indicated, but few studies on long-term follow-up have been published. Acute plantar plate rupture without structural deformity at the interphalangeal joint(s) can be ameliorated with primary PPR and flexor tendon transfer in isolation. However, in the presence of structural deformity at the level of the interphalangeal joint(s), isolated plantar plate repair is vulnerable to failure. In those circumstances, plantar plate repair combined with interphalangeal joint arthroplasty/arthrodesis, flexor tendon transfer, K-wire transfixation across the MTPJ, decompressional metatarsal shortening osteotomy, and/or concomitant procedures to restore first ray sufficiency (when indicated) are appropriate. Given that the postoperative protocols vary with the type of surgical correction, patients should be counseled accordingly. In particular, PPR and ancillary procedures such as lesser metatarsal cylindrical shortening osteotomy and/or Lapidus arthrodesis may require a longer period of a non–weight-bearing protocol and convalescence than simple arthroplasty alone. After PIPJ arthrodesis or arthroplasty, patients are permitted to be full weight-bearing in a postoperative shoe or removable cast boot unless ancillary procedures dictate differently.

ACKNOWLEDGMENTS

The author thanks librarians Lynn VanHouten and Janice Murray for their efforts and due diligence. The author also wishes to thank Dr Ninveh Hiskail for her exceptional editorial contributions.

REFERENCES

1. McGlamry ED, Jimenez AL, Green DR. Lesser ray deformities, Part 1: deformities of the intermediate digits and the metatarsophalangeal joint. In: Banks AS, Downey MS, Martin DE, et al, editors. McGlamry's comprehensive textbook of foot and ankle surgery. 3rd edition. Philadelphia: Lippincott Williams & Wilkins; 2001. p. 253–304.
2. Coughlin MJ. Lesser-toe abnormalities. J Bone Joint Surg Am 2002;84:1446–69.
3. Hansen ST. The dysfunctional forefoot. In Functional reconstruction of the foot and ankle. Philadelphia: Lippincott Williams & Wilkins; 2000. p. 215–26.
4. Yu GV, Judge MS, Hudson JR, et al. Predislocation syndrome: progressive subluxation/dislocation of the lesser metatarsophalangeal joint. J Am Podiatr Med Assoc 2002;92:182–99.
5. Bouche RT, Heit EJ. Combined plantar plate and hammertoe repair with flexor digitorum longus tendon transfer for chronic, severe, sagittal plane instability of the lesser metatarsophalangeal joints: preliminary observations. J Foot Ankle Surg 2008;47:125–37.
6. Silfverskiold N. Reduction of the uncrossed two-joint muscles of the leg to one-joint muscles in spastic conditions. Acta Chir Scand 1924;56:315–30.
7. Blitz NM, Ford LA, Christensen JC. Second metatarsophalangeal joint arthrography: a cadaveric correlation study. J Foot Ankle Surg 2004;43:231–40.
8. O'Kane C, Kilmartin T. Review of proximal interphalangeal joint excisional arthroplasty for the correction of second hammer toe deformity in 100 cases. Foot Ankle Int 2005;26:320–5.
9. Ford LA, Collins KB, Christensen JC. Stabilization of the subluxed second metatarsophalangeal joint: flexor tendon transfer versus primary repair of the plantar plate. J Foot Ankle Surg 1998;37:217–22.
10. Blitz NM, Ford LA, Christensen JC. Plantar plate repair of the second metatarsophalangeal joint: technique and tips. J Foot Ankle Surg 2004;43:266–70.
11. Coughlin MJ, Dorris J, Polk E. Operative repair of fixed hammertoe deformity. Foot Ankle Int 2000;21:94–104.
12. Dhukaram V, Hossain S, Sampath J, et al. Correction of hammer toe with an extended release of the metatarsophalangeal joint. J Bone Joint Surg Br 2002; 84:986–90.
13. Monson DK, Buell TR, Scurran BL. Lesser digital arthrodesis. Clin Podiatr Med Surg 1986;3:347–56.
14. Schlefman BS, Fenton CS, Mcglamry ED. Peg in hole arthrodesis. J Am Podiatry Assoc 1983;73:187–95.
15. Miller JM, Blacklidge DK, Ferdowsian V, et al. Chevron arthrodesis of the interphalangeal joint for hammertoe correction. J Foot Ankle Surg 2010;49:194–6.
16. Lemm M, Green R, Green D. Summary of retrospective long-term review of proximal interphalangeal joint arthroplasty and arthrodesis procedures for hammertoe correction. In: Miller SJ, Mahan KT, Yu GV, et al, editors. Reconstructive surgery of the foot and leg – update, vol. 96. Tucker (GA): The Podiatry Institute; 1996. p. 193–6.
17. Lamm BM, Ribeiro CE, Vlahovic TC, et al. Lesser proximal interphalangeal joint arthrodesis: a retrospective analysis of the peg-in-hole and end-to-end procedures. J Am Podiatr Med Assoc 2001;91:331–6.
18. Alvine FG, Garvin KL. Peg and dowel fusion of the proximal interphalangeal joint. Foot Ankle 1980;1:90–4.
19. Creighton RE, Blustein SM. Buried Kirschner wire fixation in digital fusion. J Foot Ankle Surg 1995;34:567–70.

20. Konkel KF, Sover ER, Menger AG, et al. Hammer toe correction using an absorbable pin. Foot Ankle Int 2011;32(10):973–8.
21. Soule RE. Operation for the cure of hammertoe. New York Medical Journal 1910; 91:649–52.
22. Harris W, Mote GA, Malay DS. Fixation of the proximal interphalangeal arthrodesis with the use of an intraosseous loop of stainless-steel wire suture. J Foot Ankle Surg 2009;48:411–4.
23. Caterini R, Farsetti P, Tarantino U, et al. Arthrodesis of the toe joints with an intramedullary cannulated screw for correction of hammertoe deformity. Foot Ankle Int 2004;25:256–61.
24. Baig AU, Geary NP. Fusion rate and patient satisfaction in proximal interphalangeal joint fusion of the minor toes using Kirschner wire fixation. Foot 1996;6: 120–1.
25. Reece AT, Stone MH, Young AB. Toe fusing using Kirschner wire. A study of the postoperative infection rate and related problems. J R Coll Surg Edinb 1987;32: 158–9.
26. Deland JT, Lee K, Sobel M, et al. Anatomy of the plantar plate and its attachments in the lesser metatarsal phalangeal joint. Foot Ankle Int 1995;16:480–6.
27. Johnston RB III, Smith J, Daniels T. The plantar plate of the lesser toes: an anatomical study in human cadavers. Foot Ankle Int 1994;15:276–82.
28. Lui TH, Chan LK, Chan KB. Modified plantar plate tenodesis for correction of claw toe deformity. Foot Ankle Int 2010;31(7):584–91.
29. Powless SH, Elze ME. Metatarsophalangeal joint capsular tears: an analysis by arthrography, a new classification system and surgical management. J Foot Ankle Surg 2001;40:374–89.

Early Weightbearing of the Lapidus Bunionectomy: Is it Feasible?

Neal M. Blitz, DPM

KEYWORDS

- Lapidus bunionectomy • Early weightbearing • Nonunion • Fusion

KEY POINTS

- Early weightbearing of the Lapidus bunionectomy in now mainstreamed.
- Studies with early weightbearing protocols demonstrate fusion rates equivalent or better than nonweightbearing protocols.
- Early weightbearing protocols vary and include immediate weightbearing in a postoperative shoe, partial weightbearing in a cam walker, and a period of nonweightbearing to allow for soft tissue healing then protected weightbearing.
- Potential poor candidates for early weightbearing are smokers, neuropathics, and osteoporotic patients.
- A stable fixation construct is critical when considering an early weightbearing program.
- Modern third-generation Lapidus plating systems are designed to support significant loads and contoured specifically for the first tarsometatarsal joint anatomy.

The Lapidus procedure is no longer considered a strict nonweightbearing bunionectomy.[1–12] Rigid internal fixation has provided stability of the fusion construct, allowing surgeons to mobilize patients sooner than traditionally thought.[2,3] Studies have emerged demonstrating that early weightbearing programs achieve fusion rates equivalent or better than nonweightbearing protocols.[1,4–9] The orthopedic industry has also recognized this shift and produced specialized plating systems to provide additional and alternative fixation options.

WHAT IS A LAPIDUS BUNIONECTOMY EARLY WEIGHTBEARING PROGRAM?

Early weightbearing refers to allowing patients to place weight on their operative extremity before boney consolidation of the fusion (a process that takes 6–8 weeks).

Disclosures: The author is a consultant to Orthofix, Inc., and receives royalties for the Orthofix Contours Lapidus Plating System.
Department of Orthopaedic Surgery, Bronx-Lebanon Hospital Center, Albert Einstein College of Medicine, 1650 Grand Concourse, 7th Floor, Bronx, NY 10457, USA
E-mail address: nealblitz@gmail.com

Clin Podiatr Med Surg 29 (2012) 367–381
doi:10.1016/j.cpm.2012.04.009
0891-8422/12/$ – see front matter
podiatric.theclinics.com

There are no rigid guidelines for the amount of weight allowance and at what point after the index operation patients can begin this process.

Time to Initiate Early Weightbearing Protocol

Some recommend a period of nonweightbearing for 2 weeks after the surgery to allow for soft tissue healing.[1] Others allow immediate weightbearing as tolerated.[6] Nonetheless, each surgeon has their own protocols based on their experiences and comfort level. As surgeons continue to use early weightbearing programs and have satisfactory results, protocols continue to advance.

Type of Extrinsic Protection

The fusion site still needs to be supported extrinsically during the postoperative healing process. Surgeons have used weightbearing short leg casts, removable walking boots, and postoperative shoes. A cast provides the most amount of protection.[10] A removable boot allows for patients to specifically exercise the foot and ankle. A postoperative shoe provides the least extrinsic support, and surgeons should be confident that the internal fixation is stable enough to support the loads of weightbearing when choosing this method.

Amount of Weight Allowance

The amount of weight that a patient can place postoperatively is also not clearly delineated. Some advocate gradual increases in weightbearing pressure over the course of 6 weeks, whereas others allow immediate weightbearing. Proper patient selection and fixation method are probably the most critical factors when selecting patients suitable for a postoperative weightbearing program after Lapidus bunionectomy.[1,2]

THE STIGMA OF NONUNION WITH POSTOPERATIVE WEIGHTBEARING

Early experience with the Lapidus procedure resulted in a nonunion rate up to 25%, and this was a major deterrent to surgeons performing the Lapidus procedure.[3] Postoperative weightbearing was inappropriately blamed as the cause of the nonunions, and it was not until experience with the Lapidus that poor inadequate nonrigid fixation was demonstrated to be the cause of the high nonunions seen in the early part of the century.

Dr Paul Lapidus also experienced this high nonunion rate (in the 1930s) because the fixation method of choice was suture.[13–15] Screw fixation was introduced in the 1970s and surgeons started performing the procedure with more regularity in the 1980s.[10,11,16] Screw fixation provided stability of the fusion, allowing for more reliable and acceptable fusion rates (**Figs. 1** and **2**).

Experience and better fixation methods have brought the nonunion rate to 3% to 12% of cases, a more palatable number for surgeons.[17–24] Recent studies have suggested that the nonunion rate is even lower in 0% to 5.3% of cases.[1,25] Nonunions exists even in the best hands and for the most part should not be considered a complication, but rather an expected outcome in a low percentage of cases.

There are patient and surgeon factors that can contribute to nonunion occurrence. Surgeons should be mindful of the technical aspects of the procedure and chose a stable fixation method to decrease the possibility of nonunion. Nonetheless, some patients are predisposed to bone healing difficulties because of genetic factors, medical comorbidities, and habits (ie, smoking) (**Fig. 3**). Furthermore, nonunions may be asymptomatic (not painful) and should be considered a radiographic finding.

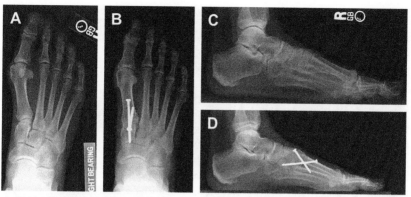

Fig. 1. Screw fixation of the Lapidus bunionectomy with two-crossed screws. (*A, C*) Preoperative weightbearing radiographs. (*B, D*) Postoperative weightbearing radiographs at 2 weeks after index operation. The first metatarsal is placed parallel to the second metatarsal, and the first metatarsal is relocated back over the sesamoids.

LITERATURE AND EARLY WEIGHTBEARING LAPIDUS

Although early weightbearing seems like a new concept, it is not. Lapidus's postoperative protocol was weightbearing in postoperative shoe with a medial plate.[13-15] Fixation options were limited at that time to support early weightbearing. However, because rigid internal fixation was introduced in the late 1980s for Lapidus arthrodesis there have been numerous studies demonstrating that early weightbearing is an acceptable postoperative protocol.[1,4-12] Between 1987 and 1992, only four studies regarding early weightbearing were produced. There was a lag of 17 years before the next wave of publications emerged and surgeons became comfortable with the procedure and improved techniques. Between 1992 and the present, seven publications demonstrate a variety of postoperative early weightbearing protocols with satisfactory results.

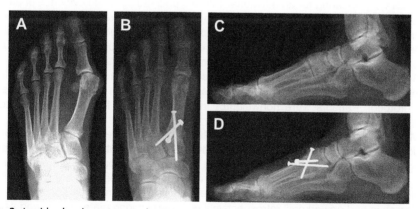

Fig. 2. Lapidus bunionectomy using two screws across the first tarsometatarsal (TMT) joint. A temporary screw into the intermediate cuneiform provides additional stability to the construct during the healing process. (*A, C*) Preoperative weightbearing radiographs. (*B, D*) Postoperative weightbearing radiographs demonstrating healed fusion. (*From* Blitz NM. The versatility of the Lapidus arthrodesis. Clin Podiatr Med Surg 2009;26:427–41.)

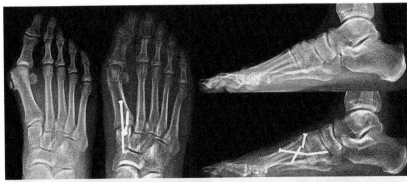

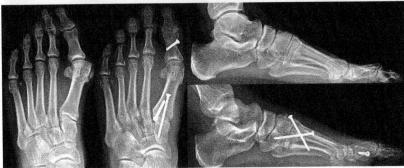

Fig. 3. Bilateral nonunion of the first TMT in a nonsmoker. This patient's surgeries were performed 8 months apart and the same technique and fixation construct were used. In some cases, patients are simply prone to nonunion.

Sangeorzan and Hansen[10] retrospectively reviewed Lapidus procedures with crossed screw fixation and an early weightbearing program in 40 feet. Their protocol involved immediate toe touch weightbearing in a short leg cast for 2 weeks. Patients were then allowed "weight of leg ambulation" for an additional 2 weeks in the cast, then full weightbearing for an additional 4 weeks until radiographic evidence of union was identified. Radiographic union was achieved in 92%. Three patients underwent revision for nonunion. Using the same postoperative early weightbearing protocol discussed previously, Clark and coworkers[11] evaluated the Lapidus arthrodesis in an adolescent population (average age of 18) in 32 feet. Fusion rate was 100%.

Bednarz and Manoli[26] performed a consecutive review of 31 feet after Lapidus arthrodeses with screw fixation. A 100% union rate was seen in their early weightbearing protocol. Patients were nonweightbearing for 2 weeks followed by protected weightbearing for 2 to 6 weeks.

Myerson and colleagues[12] evaluated 67 feet after a first metatarsocuneiform joint fusion. Twenty-one feet were placed in a short leg cast and crutches until comfortable weightbearing was tolerated. The remaining 46 feet were ambulating in a postoperative shoe with or without crutches for a duration of 6 to 8 weeks. There were seven radiographic nonunions (9.5%) and only one patient underwent a revision fusion.

Sorensen and coworkers[8] retrospectively reviewed locking plate fixation and early weightbearing. Fusion rate was 100%, and the average time to radiographic fusion was 6.95 weeks with an average time to ambulation of 2 weeks.

Kazzaz and Singh[7] allowed postoperative weightbearing in a postoperative shoe in 27 feet and achieved a successful fusion in 6 to 24 weeks, in a retrospective review.

The authors attributed the success to modern techniques of minimal bone resection, meticulous bone surface preparation, and rigid internal fixation.

Saxena and coworkers[9] performed a retrospective comparison of outcomes of Lapidus following cross screw fixation versus locking plate with screw fixation in 40 patients. The locking plate group was allowed full weightbearing at 4 weeks, whereas the screw fixation group was allowed at 6 weeks. There were no differences in postoperative complications between the two groups, and the locking plate Lapidus allowed for earlier weightbearing.

Basile and colleagues[6] retrospectively reviewed immediate weightbearing after modified Lapidus arthrodesis when two screws and a neutralization K-wire fixation were performed in 41 patients. They compared an early weightbearing protocol (immediate partial weightbearing in a removable boot) with a nonweightbearing protocol (short leg cast for 6 weeks postoperatively). No nonunions were identified and the authors suggested that a "third point of fixation may enable immediate protected weight bearing, by minimizing load placed on the crossed lag screw construct, in patients undergoing modified Lapidus arthrodesis."

In a multicenter review of 80 feet, Blitz and colleagues[1] retrospectively reviewed an early weightbearing protocol with screw fixation (two to three screws). All patients were allowed protected weightbearing after the first postoperative visit. All 80 feet proceeded to successful union (100% union), and the mean time to union was 44.5 days. Patients began protected weightbearing at a mean 14.8 days postoperative.

DeVries and colleagues[5] performed a retrospective comparison of screw fixation versus plate fixation in 143 Lapidus tarsometatarsal (TMT) joint arthrodesis. Time to full weightbearing and union rate demonstrated statistically significant improvement ($P<.001$) when locking plates were used. Locking plate and early weightbearing demonstrated a 98.5% union rate.

Menke and colleagues[4] retrospectively reviewed an early weightbearing program in 21 Lapidus fusions with locking plate combined with a single interpositional screw. Successful fusion was achieved in 90.5% and the mean time to weightbearing was 4.7 weeks.

WHICH PATIENTS ARE CANDIDATES FOR AN EARLY WEIGHTBEARING PROGRAM?

There are no exact guidelines that indicate which patients should be enrolled in an early weightbearing program. Surgeons should evaluate patients on a case-by-case basis, based on age and activity; general health status; medical comorbidities; medications; weight (body mass index); and smoking use.

Age and medical comorbidities play an important role in a patient's ability to obtain a solid union. Patients who have medical comorbidities that might affect bone healing are poor candidates. Age is not particularly a contraindication for early weightbearing so long as the patient does not have osteoporosis, which may make interfere with obtaining rigid fixation.

Obese patients can transmit excess weight onto their fusion leading to fixation failure, and increasing the chances for nonunion. Similarly, patients with peripheral neuropathy can transmit high loads to the fusion site. Smokers are well known to develop nonunions and surgeons should carefully consider early weightbearing protocols if patients cannot cease smoking.

TECHNICAL PEARLS WHEN PERFORMING A LAPIDUS BUNIONECTOMY

A curvilinear incision is most commonly used. The incision is placed dorsomedially over the first ray. The medial dorsal cuneiform nerve should specially be identified, mobilized, and protected throughout the case (**Fig. 4**).

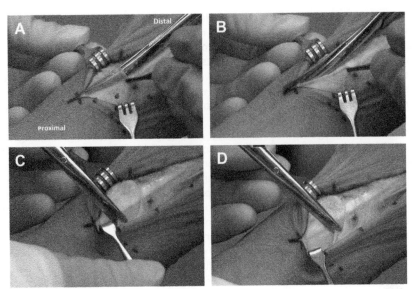

Fig. 4. Technique for protecting and retracting the medial dorsal cutaneous nerve. (*A*) The medial dorsal cutaneous nerve (*purple arrowheads*) is identified and its anatomic course is appreciated. Dissecting with a Metzenbaum scissor allows for a close inspection of the deep fascia, so that the nerve is not transected. (*B*) The deep fascia should be transected parallel to the nerve. (*C, D*) Transecting adherent bands of deep fascia allowing for the nerve to be mobilized and protected.

A concomitant McBride procedure should be performed before the midfoot fusion. Medial eminence resection and an adductor release are performed by method of choice dictated by the surgeon. However, it is important to preserve the plantar medial sagittal groove of the first metatarsal head because it limits medial and varus migration of the tibial sesamoid.

Access to the first TMT joint is achieved by a linear capsulotomy, located dorsal medially on the joint (**Fig. 5**). The author prefers the curettage method of resecting the joint, followed by perforation of the subchondral plate.

The final position of the first ray requires that the surgeon balance the metatarsal position in all three planes: transverse, sagittal, and coronal. The intermetatarsal angle should be as close to zero degrees as possible. In the sagittal plane, the first metatarsal is translated inferiorly (or plantarflexed) to accommodate the shortening that occurs when the joint is resected. The author prefers inferior translation to plantarflexion. In the coronal plane, the position should be neutral with the sesamoids relocated beneath the metatarsal head. The position of the first ray is stabilized with a K-wire before definitive fixation. Fixation can be with screws or specialized plating systems.

CAUSES OF IATROGENIC LAPIDUS NONUNION

Iatrogenic nonunion is the result of two factors: poor technique or poor fixation. Although the risk of nonunion will never cease to exist, surgeons should attempt to limit iatrogenic causes.

Preparation of the joint surface varies from surgeon to surgeon, and there is not a single way to do this, except that adequate resection of the articular cartilage must occur. The medial cuneiform and the first metatarsal base must be meticulously

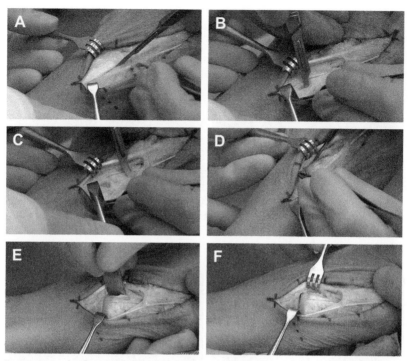

Fig. 5. Access to the first TMT joint. (*A*) A dorsal medial linear capsulotomy is made directly over the first TMT joint, and medial to the extensor hallucis longus tendon. (*B, C*) The medial capsule/periosteum is sharply reflected. (*D*) The lateral capsule is reflected distal to the joint. (*E*) Blunt dissection is performed laterally to avoid transecting any interspace vasculature. (*F*) The first TMT joint is fully exposed and ready for articular cartilage resection.

denuded of cartilage and the subchondral plate perforated to allow for bleeding bone at the interface of the fusion. Two techniques for joint preparation are "curettage resection" or "saw resection." Studies have not been performed to evaluate the effectiveness of one technique over another in terms of fusion rate.

The curettage resection involves using osteotomes or currettes to denude the cartilage, but leaves the subchondral plate intact. The subchondral plate offers some stability of the fusion site.[27] With the saw resection the entire joint and portions of the subchondral plate are resected with an oscillating saw. Thermal necrosis of the bone may occur and copious irrigation is encouraged to decrease this occurrence.

Perforation of the subchondral plate is necessary for osseous ingrowth that leads to fusion. Techniques include drilling, burring, fish scaling, and picking. When perforating the plate with a drill (or K-wire) it is important to limit thermal necrosis of bone by copious irrigation (**Fig. 6**). A bone pick may also be used without the risk of heat generation (**Fig. 7**).

Poor fixation refers to nonrigid internal fixation. According to Arbeitsgemeinschaft für Osteosynthesefragen (AO) principles, at least two points of fixation should be used. Kirschner wires do not offer compression and are not suitable for Lapidus fusion as the only method of fixation. When screws are used, at least two screws should be used. In some situations adding a third screw from the base of the first metatarsal to the second metatarsal or intermediate cuneiform provides additional stability to the construct. Surgeons should attempt to achieve compression across the fusion site.

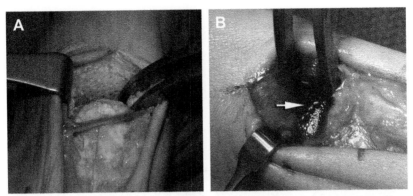

Fig. 6. Perforation of the subchondral plate. (*A*) Drilling of the subchondral plate allows for osseous ingrowth. (*B*) Fat globules (*arrow*) within the irrigation fluid indicate that the subchondral plate was appropriately perforated.

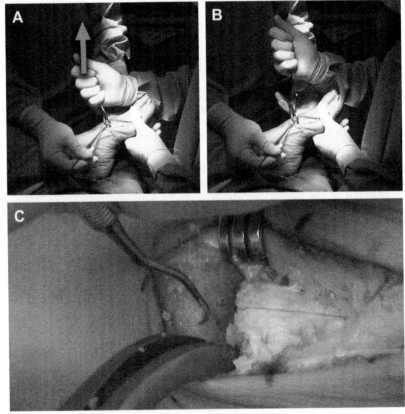

Fig. 7. Additional perforation of the subchondral plate. (*A*, *B*) Scoring of the subchondral plate with a bone pick is another way to promote perforation of the subchondral without generating heat. The technique calls for pulling of the bone pick in an upward fashion, creating ridges into the plate. (*C*) Close-up view illustrates how the subchondral plate should look when the joint preparation is complete.

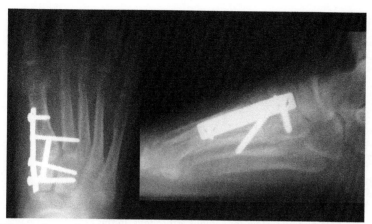

Fig. 8. Tubular plating for Lapidus. In this example, a 1.3 tubular plating system was used for Lapidus arthrodesis. Because of the limited screw options into the medial cuneiform (and the linear orientation), the screws were placed into the intermediate cuneiform for additional fixation. Similarly, a screw was placed into the second metatarsal for similar stability reasons. An isolated screw (not incorporated to the plate) traverses the fusion site. (*Courtesy of* Dr Lawrence DiDomenico, Youngstown, OH.)

Compression staples have been used and offer advantages versus simple bone staples. Plating system may be used in isolation or in conjunction with screws.

TO PLATE OR NOT TO PLATE THE LAPIDUS?

Successful clinical fusion can be achieved with screws or plates, but the ideal fixation method has yet to be determined.[28,29] Plating systems have evolved from simple tubular plates to specialty plates dedicated for the Lapidus.

First experience with plates involved linear tubular plates, which were mainly used as a bailout option when screws failed intraoperatively (**Fig. 8**). Although the linear

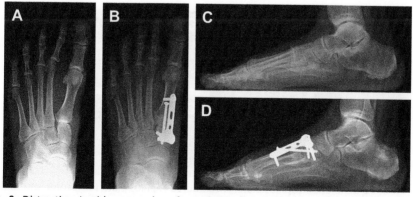

Fig. 9. Distraction Lapidus procedure for arthritic first TMT joint using a T-plate. (*A, C*) Preoperative weightbearing radiographs. Arthritic first TMT joint with long second metatarsal. (*B, D*) Postoperative healed weightbearing radiographs. In this case, a T-plate and screw that is not incorporated into the plate is used in the "belt and suspenders" fashion. This plate is not anatomic and bent to attempt to decrease its profile. (*From* Blitz NM. The versatility of the Lapidus arthrodesis. Clin Podiatr Med Surg 2009;26:427–41.)

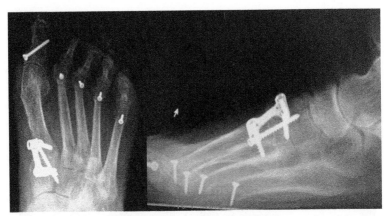

Fig. 10. Four-hole plating system for Lapidus arthrodesis. In this case the plate was used as a buttress plate, in conjunction with an isolated screw traversing the first TMT. (*Courtesy of* Dr Armol Saxena, Palo Alto, CA.)

plates offered some stability, they did not fit the area properly (especially at the medial cuneiform) and the plate could overhang into the naviculocuneiform joint. These plates needed significant bending to achieve an adequate fit but invariably fit poorly. An advantage of linear plates is the long lever arm onto the metatarsal that provides resistance to the cantilever forces that act to distract the fusion site. General T-shaped plates were also tried but did not match the shape of the medial cunieform, and the screw position was subsequently less than ideal for the medial cuneiform (**Fig. 9**). Because the T-plate has so much bulk on the medial cuneiform side, these plates invaded the anatomic insertion and course of the tibialis anterior insertion. Some surgeons used concomitant screws to provide this extra stability in a "belt and suspenders" approach.

The first generation of dedicated TMT plating systems provided a four-hole construct with two screws on both sides of the joint (**Fig. 10**). Some plates have step offs to achieve

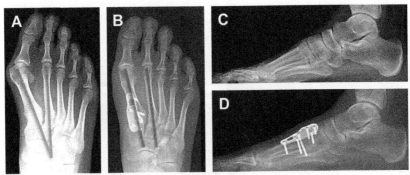

Fig. 11. Third-generation Lapidus plate. A contoured Lapidus plate for fixation of the first TMT joint (Contours Lapidus Plating System; Orthofix Inc, McKinney, TX, USA). (*A, C*) Preoperative weightbearing radiographs. (*B, D*) Weightbearing radiographs demonstrating healed fusion in anatomic position. Plating system provides three-screw hole options in the medial cuneiform, and three-screw hole options in the first metatarsal. The compression slot screw is removed intraoperatively after the compression is achieved. (*Courtesy of* Dr Neal Blitz, Bronx, NY.)

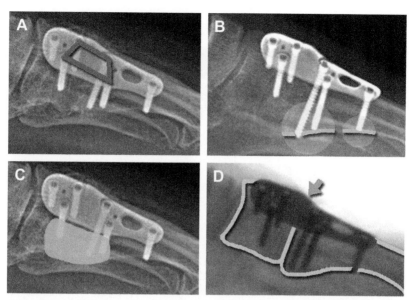

Fig. 12. Unique design features of the Contours Lapidus Plating System. (*A*) Trapezoidal periarticular screw arrangement to resist tensile loads. (*B*) Targeted locking screws are optimally placed to engage the plantar aspect of the metatarsal to resist the cantilever distracting forces. Cortical screw threads engage the plantar cortical bone (*highlighted area*). (*C*) The tibialis anterior tendon inserts on the plantarmedial aspect of the first TMT (*highlighted green area*). The plate does not interfere with the tendinous insertion. (*D*) The plate is contoured for the first TMT anatomy. A notch of the plate (*blue arrow*) is molded for the medial cuneiform, and incorporating the final position of the fusion site with the metatarsal inferiorly translated. (*Courtesy of* Dr Neal Blitz, Bronx, NY.)

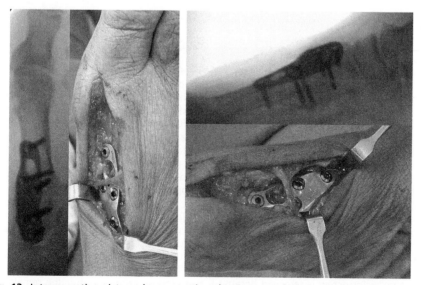

Fig. 13. Intraoperative picture demonstrating the Contoured Plating System matching the anatomy of the first TMT joint. Corresponding intraoperative fluoroscan demonstrating screw placement. One can see how this plate is contoured to the geography of the medial cuneiform and the first metatarsal base. (*Courtesy of* Dr Neal Blitz, Bronx, NY.)

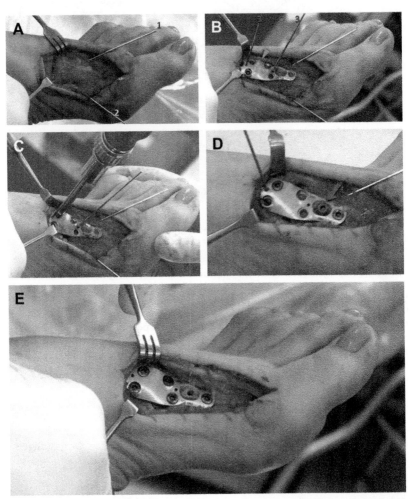

Fig. 14. Intraoperative technique for application of Contoured Plating System. (*A*) The fusion site is properly positioned. Two K-wires maintain the position, and it is important the K-wires are not placed on the dorsomedial surface because this is where the plate is placed. The first K-wire (*blue #1*) traverses the fusion site, and is placed from dorsal and lateral on the first metatarsal to plantar medial in the medial cuneiform. The second K-wire (*yellow #2*) is placed from the plantar medial base of the first metatarsal into the intermediate cuneiform. (*B*) The contoured plate is placed on the dorsal medial surface of the fusion site. A notch on the plate (*green arrowhead*) corresponds with geographic anatomy of the medial cuneiform, allowing for proper plate placement. The third K-wires (*red #3*) placed hold the plate steady. (*C*) The first screw to be placed is into the medial cuneiform. This secures the proximal aspect of the plate, allowing for the compression screw to be placed in the compression slot. (*D*) A screw is placed in the compression hole (*purple arrow*), allowing for compression to occur at the fusion site. Take note that the K-wire (*#2*) was removed before placing the compression screw to allow for uniform compression across the first TMT. (*E*) Image demonstrating all screws placed into the contoured locking plate. The compression screw is removed because it is no longer necessary after the remaining holes are filled with locking screws. (*Courtesy of* Dr Neal Blitz, Bronx, NY.)

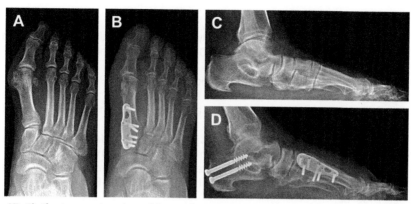

Fig. 15. Flatfoot reconstruction with Lapidus procedure (using contoured plate), calcaneal osteotomy, and posterior tibial tendon repair with flexor digitroum longus transfer. (*A, C*) Preoperative radiographs. (*B, D*) Postoperative radiographs demonstrating healed fusion. (*Courtesy of* Dr Neal Blitz, Bronx, NY.)

a better fit, and understanding the final metatarsal position is not congruent with the medial cuneiform. Locking plates offered a more stable construct. One disadvantage of a periarticular plating system, however, is that the cantilever forces are not specifically addressed within the structure of the plate and compression of the fusion site.

The second generation involved more anatomically geared locking plating systems that had a T-shape to match the limited fixation options available at the cuneiform and provide a longer metatarsal arm for a compression slot. Some surgeons use a screw not incorporated into the plate, most probably because of previous plate generation habits. One plate system offers a transfixation screw incorporated into the plate, but requires the undersurface of bone to be bored out potentially limiting the amount of bone available for fusion. These plates are also flat, and require bending to match the shape of the fusion site.

The third-generation Lapidus plating system incorporates features of previous generations, but is specially designed (contoured) for the anatomy of the fusion site (**Figs. 11–13**). The Contours Lapidus Plating System is anatomic for the first TMT; fits between the tibialis anterior insertion (inferiorly) and the extensor tendons (superiorly); and is contoured specifically for the underlying geography of the medial cuneiform and metatarsal. The medial cuneiform surface is maximized for screw options. This particular plating system design incorporates periarticular locking screws in a trapezoidal fashion, and a long metatarsal component to resist the cantilever forces. Compression is achieved with a dedicated compression hole (**Fig. 14**). Lastly, the plate design and screw position and angles incorporate the final position (shortening and inferior translation) of the fusion site. Plating systems can be used for isolated Lapidus bunionectomy or as part of a larger reconstructive foot surgery (**Fig. 15**).

SUMMARY

The Lapidus procedure should no longer be considered a strict nonweightbearing bunionectomy. In the past few years, several studies have emerged demonstrating that early weightbearing after a Lapidus fusion is indeed possible with satisfactory fusion rates. This is mainly because of improved fixation techniques available today that have allowed for better stabilization of the fusion site. Surgeons should still properly indicate patients for early weightbearing protocols.

REFERENCES

1. Blitz NM, Lee T, Williams K, et al. Early weight bearing after modified Lapidus arthodesis: a multicenter review of 80 cases. J Foot Ankle Surg 2010;49(4): 357–62.
2. Blitz NM. Early weightbearing of the Lapidus: is it possible? Podiatr Today 2004;17: 46–52.
3. Blitz NM. The versatility of the Lapidus arthrodesis. Clin Podiatr Med Surg 2009; 26:427–41.
4. Menke CR, McGlamry MC, Camasta CA. Lapidus arthrodesis with a single lag screw and a locking H-plate. J Foot Ankle Surg 2011;50(4):377–82.
5. DeVries JG, Granata JD, Hyer CF. Fixation of first tarsometatarsal arthrodesis: a retrospective comparative cohort of two techniques. Foot Ankle Int 2011; 32(2):158–62.
6. Basile P, Cook EA, Cook JJ. Immediate weight bearing following modified Lapidus arthrodesis. J Foot Ankle Surg 2010;49(5):459–64.
7. Kazzaz S, Singh D. Postoperative cast necessity after a Lapidus arthrodesis. Foot Ankle Int 2009;30(8):746–51.
8. Sorensen MD, Hyer CF, Berlet GC. Results of Lapidus arthrodesis and locked plating with early weightbearing. Foot Ankle Spec 2009;2(5):227–33.
9. Saxena A, Nguyen A, Nelsen E. Lapidus bunionectomy: early evaluation of crossed lag screws versus locking plate with plantar lag screw. J Foot Ankle Surg 2009;48(2):170–9.
10. Sangeorzan B, Hansen S. Modified Lapidus procedure for hallux valgus. Foot Ankle 1989;9:262–6.
11. Clark HR, Veith RG, Hansen ST Jr. Adolescent bunions treated by the modified Lapidus procedure. Bull Hosp Jt Dis Orthop Inst 1987;47:109–22.
12. Myerson M, Allon S, McGarvey W. Metatarsocuneiform arthrodesis for management of hallux valgus and metatarsus primus varus. Foot Ankle 1992;13:107–15.
13. Lapidus PW. Operative correction of the metatarsus varus primus in hallux valgus. Surg Gynec Obst 1934;58:183–91.
14. Lapidus PW. A quarter century of experience with the operative correction of the metatarsus varus in hallux valgus. Bull Hosp Joint Dis Orthop Inst 1956;17: 404–21.
15. Lapidus PW. The author's bunion operation from 1931 to 1959. Clin Orthop 1960; 16:119–35.
16. Rutherford R. The Lapidus procedure for primus metatarsus adductus. J Am Podiatry Assoc 1974;64:581–4.
17. Hansen ST. Functional reconstruction of the foot and ankle. Philadelphia: Lippincott Williams & Wilkins; 2000.
18. Catanzariti AR, Mendicino RW, Lee MS, et al. The modified Lapidus arthrodesis: a retrospective analysis. J Foot Ankle Surg 1999;38:322–32.
19. Kopp FJ, Patel MM, Levine DS, et al. The modified Lapidus procedure for hallux valgus: a clinical and radiographic analysis. Foot Ankle Int 2005;26:913–7.
20. Rink-Brüne O. Lapidus arthrodesis for management of hallux valgus: a retrospective review of 106 cases. J Foot Ankle Surg 2004;43:290–5.
21. Coetzee JC, Wickum D. The Lapidus procedure: a prospective cohort outcome study. Foot Ankle Int 2004;25:526–31.
22. Popelka S, Vavrík P, Hromádka R, et al. Our results of the Lapidus procedure in patients with hallux valgus deformity. Acta Chir Orthop Traumatol Cech 2008;75: 271–6.

23. Hofbauer MH, Grossman JP. The Lapidus procedure. Clin Podiatr Med Surg 1996;13:485–96.
24. McInnes BD, Couche RT. Critical evaluation of the modified Lapidus procedure. J Foot Ankle Surg 2001;40:71–90.
25. Patel S, Ford LA, Hamilton GA, et al. Modified Lapidus arthrodesis: rate of nonunion in 227 cases. J Foot Ankle Surg 2004;43:37–42.
26. Bednarz PA, Manoli A. Modified Lapidus procedure for the treatment of hypermobile hallux valgus. Foot Ankle Int 2000;21:816–21.
27. Ray RG, Ching RP, Christensen JC, et al. Biomechanical analysis of the first metatarsocuneiform arthrodesis. J Foot Ankle Surg 1998;37:376–85.
28. Klos K, Gueorguiev B, Muckley T, et al. Stability of medial locking plate and compression screw versus two crossed screws for Lapidus arthrodesis. Foot Ankle Int 2010;31(2):158–63.
29. Klos K, Simons P, Hajduk AS, et al. Plantar versus dorsomedial plate for Lapidus arthrodesis: a biomechanical analysis. Foot Ankle Int 2011;32(11):1081–5.

Subtalar Arthroereisis and Its Role in Pediatric and Adult Population

Daphne Yen-Douangmala, DPM, Mher Vartivarian, DPM, J. Danny Choung, DPM*

KEYWORDS

- Subtalar arthroereisis • Flatfoot • Sinus tarsi pain

KEY POINTS

- Subtalar arthroereisis is a widely used surgical procedure that can effectively address flexible flatfoot deformities in both pediatric and adult populations.
- The advantages of subtalar arthroereisis include simplicity of surgical technique, significant deformity correction while sparing hindfoot arthrodesis or osteotomy, and brevity of non–weight bearing or protected weight bearing postoperatively.
- Because flatfoot deformity is a complicated, multidimensional structural disfigurement, subtalar arthroereisis rarely can be applied as an isolated procedure but should be adjunctive to other soft tissue and osseous procedures.
- The most common postoperative complication in both pediatric and adult populations is sinus tarsi pain.
- Explantation of the subtalar arthroereisis implant after an adequate period of time from the original surgery does not seem to result in loss of correction in the majority of pediatric and adult patients.

Subtalar joint arthroereisis is a surgical procedure that addresses symptomatic flexible flatfoot deformities, using an extra-articular implant within the sinus tarsi. Historically, the procedure has been described primarily for juvenile deformities but has been extended to address adult deformities. The implant is often referred to as internal orthotic or endo-orthotic, providing artificial support or bracing without the need of daily patient cooperation or compliance. It functions to limit pronation of the hindfoot by primarily acting at the subtalar joint, but, more importantly, improves the talar position and alignment relative to the calcaneus and navicular.[1,2]

Different implants have been developed for this procedure, which Vogler[3] classified into 3 groups: self-locking wedge, axis-altering device, and impact-blocking device. Whether or not this implant classification scheme accurately depicts the differing

Department of Podiatric Surgery, Kaiser Foundation Hospital, 99 Montecillo Road, San Rafael, CA 94903, USA
* Corresponding author.
E-mail address: dchoung@gmail.com

Clin Podiatr Med Surg 29 (2012) 383–390
doi:10.1016/j.cpm.2012.04.001
0891-8422/12/$ – see front matter © 2012 Elsevier Inc. All rights reserved.

functions of the available implants,[4] the self-locking wedge implants are the focus of this article, because they currently are the most commonly used.[5]

Various self-locking wedge implants have been developed, but they all have a threaded design and a cylindrical or conical shape. These implants are placed into the sinus tarsi and oriented toward the tarsal canal, inserted like a screw with the threads intended to engage the floor of the sinus tarsi, the leading edge of the talar body, the plantarlateral surface of the talar neck, and the interosseous talocalcaneal ligament. Discussion of subtalar arthroereisis in this article assumes this particular implant type unless otherwise stated.

BENEFITS OF ARTHROEREISIS

When appropriately executed, subtalar joint arthroereisis has the potential to significantly restore proper hindfoot anatomy in a flexible flatfoot deformity. The proposed advantages of the procedure versus other surgical methods are manifold. It is simple and quick to perform through a small incision, and the hindfoot can be spared arthrodesis or osteotomy. Recovery usually involves a brief period of non–weight bearing or protected weight bearing that is significantly less compared to most osseous procedures. These advantages are appealing to both surgeons and patients, because the procedure is perceived as a reasonably uncomplicated and efficient means of surgically correcting a flatfoot deformity.

When the procedure is applied to the juvenile flatfoot, there is the additional premise that the orthotic effect allows for favorable musculoskeletal adjustment during a child's physical maturation, which influences the foot in obtaining intrinsic stability, rendering the implant ultimately unnecessary.[6,7]

For these reasons, subtalar arthroereisis has become a prominent surgical option for flexible flatfoot correction. Despite its original emphasis on pediatric flatfoot deformities, it seems increasingly used in the adult population. It has been even further extended to treat the rigid flatfoot with talocalcaneal coalition.[8] This broad application to flatfoot deformities testifies to its perceived efficacy in addition to its simplicity. Subtalar arthroereisis, however, is not applicable to all flatfoot deformities, whether flexible or rigid, or as an isolated or adjunctive procedure. Those deformities that particularly favor transverse plane dominance may not be suited for arthroereisis. Other complex factors in flatfoot deformities, such as primary joint contribution, associated soft tissue adaptation, relative muscle function, and the presence or absence of connective tissue or neuromuscular causes, dictate judicious evaluation and surgical planning, and arthroereisis may be the least applicable or a completely ineffective procedure.

Relative contraindications reported for this procedure include flatfoot associated with angular deformity at the knee, torsional leg deformities, metatarsus adductus deformities, and valgus ankles,[9,10] whereas reported absolute contraindications include subtalar joint arthritis, peroneal muscle spasm, and excessive ligamentous laxity.[7,9,11–13]

THE ARTHROEREISIS CONTROVERSY

In spite of its wide use, there is no definitive consensus or guidelines for its use in children and adults. In regards to optimum age of application in children, Koning and colleagues[7] believe arthroereisis to have little lasting effect on children beyond age 10 and report the ideal age for arthroereisis is 8 years. Fernandez de Retana[6] and colleagues, however, advocate arthroereisis be performed before age 12, to allow a remodeling period of at least 2 years, assuming that the foot reaches its full maturity at 14 to 15 years.

In adults who already have obtained full skeletal maturity, this proposed long-term effect of subtalar arthroereisis does not pertain. Reports of retained skeletal correction in adults after explantation, however, suggest otherwise. In a prospective study, Needleman[12] proposed that implants in place for 8 months allow stiffening of the soft tissues that are integral to joint alignment and motion. This seems to be extrapolated from the finding that in those patients who required implant removal 8 or more months after the index procedure, no significant difference could be detected for the 3 radiographic parameters evaluated before and after explantation: medial longitudinal arch, uncovering of the talar head, and the difference in standing ankle height. The strength of this claim is questionable, because subtalar arthroereisis was often combined with other soft tissue or osseous procedures (eg, tendo-Achilles lengthening or gastrocnemius recession, Evans osteotomy, and/or Lapidus arthrodesis or Cotton osteotomy), which could serve as confounding variables.

Schon[13] similarly postulates that when subtalar arthroereisis is used as an adjunct procedure in conjunction with medial soft tissue stabilizing procedures, the implant typically is no longer needed after soft tissue healing and may be removed without risk to the surgical correction. This is premised on arthroereisis protecting and facilitating healing of the medial soft tissue reconstruction while concomitantly allowing progressive introduction of weight bearing without causing excessive strain on the medial ligaments and tendons.

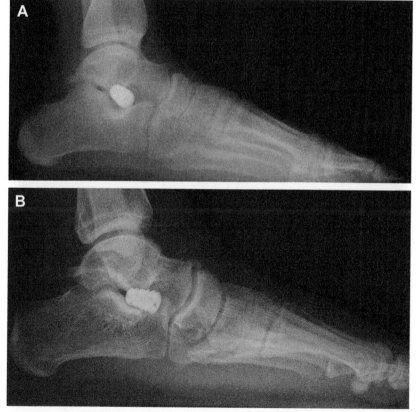

Fig. 1. A 13-year-old boy who underwent gastrocnemius recession and subtalar arthroereisis for treatment of a painful flexible flatfoot. (*A*) Postoperative weight-bearing lateral radiograph, approximately 8 weeks after surgery. (*B*) Weight-bearing lateral radiograph, 33 months after surgery. Note the anterior displacement of the implant.

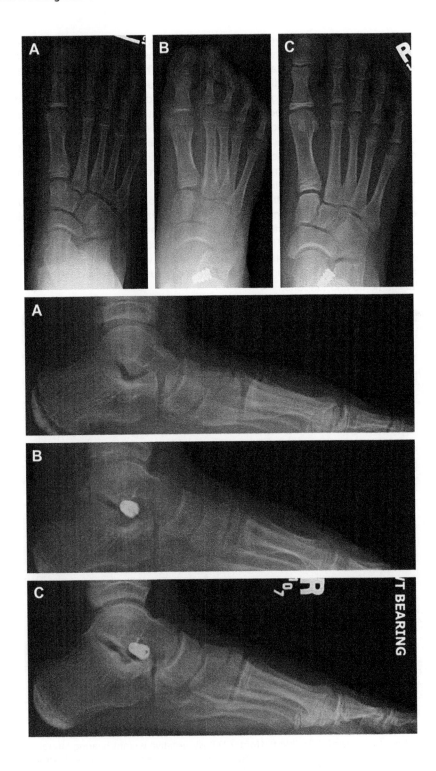

The 2005 clinical practice guidelines for adult flatfoot suggest that arthroereisis should only be used for early stage II posterior tibial tendon dysfunction or non–posterior tibial tendon dysfunction adult flexible flatfoot secondary to equinus.[14] Consistent with other literature, caution is implied in the application of arthroereisis as an isolated procedure. Long-term compensation and adaptive changes to the foot may require ancillary soft tissue or osseous procedures for appropriate medial column stabilization. Invariably, equinus needs to be surgically addressed.

In addition to flexible flatfoot deformities, subtalar joint arthroereisis has been used in the correction of rigid flatfoot deformities due to tarsal coalitions in children. Giannini and colleagues[8] reported on the outcome of coalition resection with subtalar arthroereisis in the treatment of flatfeet with talocalcaneal coalitions in 12 patients and 14 feet. Median age of the patients was 14 years (9–18 years) and median follow-up was 40 months (30–64 months). Eighty-six percent of the patients had improvement of pain, and 92.8% had improvement of subtalar joint range of motion. Three patients with fair results were the oldest of the patient population, and their outcome worsened with time. The satisfaction outcome in this study still fell within the range reported for those in pediatric flexible flatfoot deformities.[5–7] The investigators noted better results before the age of 14, which supports the assumption that the foot reaches full maturity at the age of 14 or 15 years,[6] rendering it incapable of positive adaptation and tolerance of the implant. In the context of skeletally mature pediatric population with talocalcaneal coalitions, the posterior subtalar joint is likely too maladapted for any benefit from procedures short of a subtalar joint arthrodesis. Studies that correlate the success of subtalar arthroereisis with the extent of middle facet coalition may further elucidate the utility of this procedure in these rigid disorders. Pediatric rigid flatfoot secondary to a calcaneonavicular bar may also be considered more suitable for a subtalar arthroereisis, because the subtalar joint is theoretically unaffected from this coalition.

COMPLICATIONS

Complications from the procedure seem impartial to age. The most common reported complication is sinus tarsi pain, which is directly attributed to the implant. Zaret and Myerson[15] reported sinus tarsi pain in 18% of patients. Needleman[12] reported 46% of adult patients having postoperative sinus tarsi pain. In the pediatric population, complication rates up to 29.6% have been reported.[7] Most patients seem to have resolution of pain after implant removal. In a study to identify risk factors leading to subtalar implant removal, where the mean age was 30.8 years (range 8.8–62.2 years), Cook and colleagues[16] found no difference in age between patients who required explantation and those who did not. Postoperative sinus tarsi pain has been attributed to inflammation of the soft tissues by implant placement and/or persistent strain and stress to the implant caused by unaddressed equinus.[17] In the senior author's

---

Fig. 2. Perioperative series of an 8-year-old boy who underwent gastrocnemius recession and subtalar arthroereisis. (*A*) Preoperative weight-bearing AP and lateral radiographs demonstrating flexible flatfoot deformity. (*B*) Postoperative weight-bearing AP and lateral radiographs, 1 month after surgery, demonstrates normal AP and lateral talar–first metatarsal angles and normal coverage of talar head. (*C*) Weight-bearing AP and lateral radiographs 21 months after surgery. Note the anterior displacement of implant, increased abduction of the midtarsal joint, and increased exposure of the medial talar head on the AP view. Yet, retention of corrected lateral talo–first metatarsal angle is evidenced on the lateral view.

experience, all accounts of sinus tarsi pain in the pediatric population indicated that it developed approximately 2 years after the procedure, and all were attributed to implant migration. On radiographic evaluation of each case, the implants had displaced anteriorly (**Fig. 1**). All patients had resolution of pain after explantation. Other than pain, there has been a reported case of a talar neck fracture 10 years after implantation of the Maxwell-Brancheau arthroereisis implant.[18] This supports the concern about bony remodeling or destruction from the elasticity of the implant being much stiffer than cortical bone.[17]

In the adult population, implant removal is the typical treatment for sinus tarsi pain. As discussed previously, removal does not seem to result in loss of correction in the majority of cases. Cook and colleagues[16] found that patients with a residual postoperative high transverse plane deformity, as indicated by the calcaneocuboid abduction angle, had greater odds of explantation, by 9.6%. Conversely, a smaller postoperative anteroposterior (AP) talocalcaneal angle was found protective, resulting in a 17.5% reduction in odds for explantation. It may be concluded that the flatfoot with a stronger transverse plane component may be more intolerant of the implant. These data also support the anecdotal claim that subtalar arthroereisis alone may not be appropriate for flatfoot deformities with a significant transverse plane component.[10,17,19] The senior author's experience concurs with this opinion. In the same pediatric cases that required subtalar implant removal, radiographic findings of increased AP talocalcaneal and AP talar–first metatarsal angle were found. These changes were not evident radiographically within the first 6 months after surgery but were discovered at presentation of sinus tarsi pain approximately 2 years postoperatively. The lateral talocalcaneal angle retained the original correction, however, despite implant migration and subsequent removal (**Fig. 2**).

SUMMARY

Inferences from clinical studies and anecdotal assumptions seem to agree that subtalar arthroereisis has a valid role in the surgical treatment of flexible flatfoot deformities. Subtalar arthroereisis has been used since 1946,[20] and, despite the paucity of literature, there exist varying ideas as to its indications. The gradual evolution in implant design, function, and simplicity has coincided with amplification of its usage, especially with the self-locking wedge implant. Whereas sinus tarsi implants have been regularly used for many years in European countries,[6] it recently has gained wide acceptance in the United States, with increasing interest in its application for adult-acquired flatfoot and posterior tibial tendon dysfunction. It is a procedure that contends with arthrodesis and osteotomy procedures not only because of its technical ease but also its capacity to significantly correct deformity.

The complications associated with the self-locking implants do not seem any more adverse or frequent than those associated with other osseous or soft tissue procedures. It may even be argued that less patient morbidity is associated with subtalar arthroereisis. It is an appealing procedure in that it typically spares hindfoot arthrodesis procedures in the correction of flatfoot deformities, but it should not be used to the exclusion of arthrodesis or osteotomies altogether. Most, if not all, the literature pertaining to subtalar arthroereisis promotes adjunctive soft tissue and osseous procedures.

Subtalar arthroereisis may be technically simple, but flatfoot deformities are complex in their variegated presentation. The deformity is multiplanar, typically assessed relative to the 3 cardinal planes for better comprehension, yet elusive to precise quantification relative to planar and joint dominance or contribution, soft tissue involvement, and other modifying variables. As with any other flatfoot procedure, subtalar arthroereisis should be applied as part of a surgical armamentarium in addressing a challenging, multifaceted problem that requires careful and thorough evaluation. Foot and ankle surgeons should not propose subtalar arthroereisis simply because of its ease, low morbidity, and quicker recovery time. It is rare that this procedure can be applied in isolation, especially in the adult population. In the authors' opinion, the procedure should not be construed merely as a substitute for hindfoot arthrodesis or osteotomy but as one of many surgical methods that, when appropriately applied, has the unique benefit of sparing a joint, retaining more hindfoot motion, and powerfully correcting deformity. When subtalar arthroereisis is represented in an either-or context, there is danger of shortsightedness, underappreciation of the deformity, and misapplication of the procedure.

REFERENCES

1. Christensen JC, Campbell N, Dinucci K. Closed kinetic chain tarsal mechanics of subtalar joint arthroereisis. J Am Podiatr Med Assoc 1996;86:467–73.
2. Husain ZS, Fallat LM. Biomechanical analysis of Maxwell-Brancheau Arthroereisis Implants. J Foot Ankle Surg 2002;41:352–8.
3. Vogler HW. STJ blocking operation for pathological pronation syndrome. In: McGlamry ED, editor. Comprehensive textbook of foot surgery. Baltimore (MD): Williams and Wilkins; 1987. p. 466–82.
4. Kirby KA. Understanding the biomechanics of subtalar joint arthroereisis. Podiatry Today 2011;24:36–45.
5. Highlander P, Sung W, Weil L Jr. Subtalar arthroereisis. Clin Podiatr Med Surg 2011;28:745–54.
6. Fernandez de Retana P, Alvarez F, Viladot R. Subtalar arthroereisis in pediatric flatfoot reconstruction. Foot Ankle Clin N Am 2010;15:323–35.
7. Koning PM, Heesterbeek PJ, de Visser E. Subtalar arthroereisis for pediatric flexible pes planovalgus: fifteen years experience with the cone-shaped implant. J Am Podiatr Med Assoc 2009;99:447–53.
8. Giannini S, Ceccarelli F, Vannini F, et al. Operative treatment of flatfoot with talocalcaneal coalition. Clin Orthop Relat Res 2003;411:178–87.
9. Dockery GL, Crawford MD. The Maxwell-Brancheau athroereisis (MBA) implant in pediatric and adult flexible flatfoot conditions. Foot Ankle Q 1999;12:107–20.
10. Maxwell JR, Carro A, Sun C. Use of the Maxwell-Bancheau arthroereisis implant for the correction of posterior tibial tendon dysfunction. Clin Podiatr Med Surg 1999;16:479–89.
11. Jahss MH. The subtalar complex. In: Jahss MH, editor. Disorders of the foot & ankle. 2nd edition. Philadelphia: W.B. Saunders Company; 1991. p. 1333–71.
12. Needleman RL. A surgical approach for flexible flatfeet in adults including a subtalar arthroereisis with the MBA sinus tarsi implant. Foot Ankle Int 2006;27:9.
13. Schon LC. Subtalar arthroereisis: a new exploration of an old concept. Foot Ankle Clin N Am 2007;12:329–39.
14. Lee MS, Vanore JV, Thomas JL, et al. Clinical practice guideline adult flatfoot panel. Diagnosis and treatment of adult flatfoot. J Foot Ankle Surg 2005;44:78–113.
15. Zaret DI, Myerson MS. Arthroereisis of the subtalar joint. Foot Ankle Clin 2003;8:605–17.
16. Cook EA, Cook JJ, Basile P. Identifying risk factors in subtalar arthroereisis explantation: a propensity-matched analysis. J Foot Ankle Surg 2011;50:395–401.

17. Chang TJ, Lee J. Subtalar joint arthroereisis in adult-acquired flatfoot and posterior tibial tendon dysfunction. Clin Podiatr Med Surg 2007;24:687–97.
18. Corpuz M, Shofler D, Labovitz J, et al. Fracture of the talus as a complication of subtalar arthroereisis. J Foot Ankle Surg 2012;51:91–4.
19. Soomekh DJ, Baravarian B. Pediatric and adult flatfoot reconstruction: subtalar arthroereisis versus realignment osteotomy surgical options. Clin Podiatr Med Surg 2006;223:695–708.
20. Chambers EF. An operation for the correction of flexible flat feet of adolescents. West J Surg Obstet Gynecol 1946;54:77–86.

End-Stage Ankle Arthritis
Arthrodiastasis, Supramalleolar Osteotomy, or Arthrodesis?

Lawrence A. DiDomenico, DPM[a,b,*], Nik Gatalyak, DPM[a]

KEYWORDS

• Ankle • Arthritis • Arthrodiastasis • Supramalleolar osteotomy • Arthrodesis

KEY POINTS

• End-stage ankle joint arthritis is a disabling and painful condition.
• A thorough history and physical and advanced imaging is paramount to an appropriate diagnosis of end-stage ankle arthritis.
• Osseous alignment is necessary to maintain a good long-term outcome.

INTRODUCTION

One of the most challenging issues posed to foot and ankle surgeons is whether to perform a joint-sparing or a joint-destructive procedure for patients with end-stage ankle arthritis. Even more taxing for the foot and ankle surgeon is how to treat this condition in the younger patient population, in particular patients in their 20s, 30s, and 40s.

Patients who suffer with end-stage ankle arthritis have compromised quality of life. Nonsurgical treatment should be considered before surgery. The gold standard for end-stage ankle arthritis is currently ankle arthrodesis. With the advancements of AO fixation and plating technology, ankle arthrodesis has become a time tested and predictable joint destructive procedure. For years, foot and ankle surgeons have been looking for alternatives to ankle arthrodesis. The most common alternatives currently are the joint-sparing procedures, which consist of arthrodiastasis, total ankle replacements, total ankle allograft replacement, and supramalleolar osteotomies.

With reasonable reported outcomes in the literature, ankle arthrodiastasis provides foot and ankle surgeons another procedure option. Because the newer generations of ankle implants have a better anatomic design, coupled with significant successful

[a] Reconstructive Rearfoot & Ankle Surgical Fellowship, Ankle and Foot Care Centers, Ohio College of Podiatric Medicine, 8175 Market Street, Youngstown, OH 44512, USA; [b] St. Elizabeth Hospital, Youngstown, OH, USA
* Corresponding author. Reconstructive Rearfoot & Ankle Surgical Fellowship, Ankle and Foot Care Centers, Ohio College of Podiatric Medicine, 8175 Market Street, Youngstown, OH 44512.
E-mail address: ld5353@aol.com

Clin Podiatr Med Surg 29 (2012) 391–412
doi:10.1016/j.cpm.2012.04.010
0891-8422/12/$ – see front matter © 2012 Elsevier Inc. All rights reserved.

podiatric.theclinics.com

literature review, the implants are becoming increasingly popular as an alternative to ankle arthrodesis. Although not commonly performed, total ankle allograft transplant replacement has been sporadically reported in the literature as another possible substitute to ankle fusion. Supramalleolar osteotomies are performed to realign the distal tibia and improve foot and ankle function in those patients who suffer from end-stage ankle joint arthritis and juxta-articular tibial deformity.

ARTHRITIS

Osteoarthritis is a degenerative disease of joints characterized by formation of osteophytes, subchondral sclerosis, subchondral cysts, loose bodies, and joint space narrowing.[1-3] It affects approximately 15% of the world's population, of which 1% is suffering with osteoarthritis of the ankle.[2] In the United States, arthritis is the leading cause of disability. About 21 million people reported having arthritis, and subsequent limitation of their work-related function has been found in 1 out of 3 of these people.[4] Daily function is significantly affected compared with the general population.[5] According to Glazebrook and colleagues,[3] end-stage ankle arthritis has a severe impact on pain, health-related quality of life, and function that is at least as severe as patients with end-stage hip arthritis. In general, patients with end-stage ankle arthritis experience greater emotional and mental distress than those who are experiencing end-stage hip arthritis.

The causes of osteoarthritis can be divided into 3 categories: primary, secondary, and posttraumatic. Primary osteoarthritis is idiopathic in nature with no obvious underlying abnormalities occurring 50% of the time, whereas secondary osteoarthritis occurs in patients with underlying conditions such as rheumatoid arthritis, hemarthroses, hemophilia, and postinfectious processes. Although primary osteoarthritis is the most common cause of hip and knee problems, the same is not observed in the ankle.[3,5-10] Primary osteoarthritis of the ankle affects older populations of patients. The primary group also has less pain and increased range of motion compared with secondary and posttraumatic osteoarthritis groups.[2,6,11] Valderrabano and colleagues[2] evaluated 406 ankles with symptomatic end-stage osteoarthritis. In their study, posttraumatic osteoarthritis of the ankle was seen in 78% of cases, secondary osteoarthritis in 19% of cases, and primary osteoarthritis in 9% of cases. Similar results were found by Saltzman and colleagues,[6] evaluating 639 ankles with 70% of cases occurring secondary to trauma of the ankle joint. Malleolar ankle fractures, ligamentous injuries causing ankle instability, pilon tibial fractures, tibial shaft fractures, talus fractures, osteochondritis dissecans, and severe combined fractures were the main causes of posttraumatic osteoarthritis of the ankle seen in both studies (**Fig. 1**).

NONOPERATIVE CARE

Conservative treatments are limited for symptomatic end-stage ankle arthritis. Most therapies provide short-term improvement of symptoms and should be exhausted before consideration of surgical treatment options. Nonoperative, conservative treatment options include a combination of medications, injections, modification of activities, prescription of custom orthotic devices, and bracing.[12-14]

Nonsteroidal antiinflammatory drugs (NSAIDs) may help relieve pain of arthritic ankle joints. They should be given only short term and closely monitored for side effects. Altered kidney function tests as well as bleeding tendencies are the most common side effects associated with NSAIDs. A combination of corticosteroid-anesthetic intra-articular injection can be given to decrease joint pain and inflammation. Varied results have been reported for the duration of beneficial effects of the

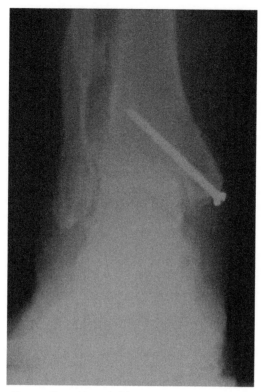

Fig. 1. End-stage posttraumatic ankle arthritis.

injection. Side effects are uncommon but skin depigmentation and infections may be seen. Modification of activities may be beneficial. Patients' pain may be more manageable with changes in occupation to a sedentary job as well as a decrease in vigorous activities such as sports. Pain and inflammation can also be managed with bracing and change in shoe gear. Rocker-bottom sole, solid ankle cushion heel (SACH), lace-up ankle support braces, ankle-foot orthosis, and weight-bearing fiberglass or plaster cast can decrease inflammation and pain by restricting motion of the ankle joint. Patella tendon–bearing (PTB) braces have also been used with some success for treatment of ankle arthritis because they reduce pain and discomfort of the affected extremity by decreasing axial load **(Fig. 2)**.[12–14]

ARTHRODIASTASIS

The term arthrodiastasis comes from the Greek words arthro (joint), dia (through), and tasis (to stretch out). Distraction of the ankle joint has been used as an alternative to arthrodesis or arthroplasty. This procedure is advocated to reduce pain and increase motion of an arthritic joint without sacrificing the joint. It is indicated in younger patients with good bone stock and painful ankle joints who are not willing to have an ankle arthrodesis.[15,16]

The technique was first described by Judet in 1978 for treatment of osteoarthritis of the hip.[17] It was not until 1995 that van Valburg and colleagues[17] reported on the use of an arthrodiastasis technique for treatment of severe posttraumatic arthritis of the ankle joint. The Ilizarov external fixator was used for ankle distraction in 11 patients

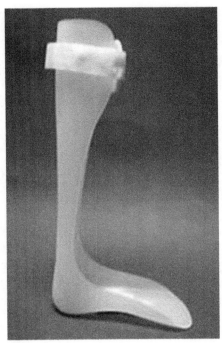

Fig. 2. An ankle-foot orthosis. This is one of many types of ankle-foot orthosis that is often used to limit the motion of the ankle joint to treat end-stage ankle joint arthritis nonoperatively.

in combination with measurement of intra-articular hydrostatic pressure. The Ilizarov external fixator was applied for 3 months and the ankle joint was distracted 5 mm. Patients were able to be fully weight bearing just days after surgery. At 3 months, the fixator was removed and patients were transitioned into a cam boot. Clinical improvement of pain and mobility was observed at mean follow-up of 20 months and an increase in joint space was also noted on weight-bearing radiographs. During loading, the researchers observed an increase in intra-articular pressures of the distracted ankles.

After distraction of a joint, theoretically the cartilage has the potential to repair itself. It is thought that mechanical off-loading can prevent further damage to the articular cartilage. Once the joint is off-loaded, the chondrocyte repair process may begin with fluctuation in intra-articular hydrostatic pressure during weight bearing with the external fixator. Chondrocytes are able to repair by the cyclic changes in intra-articular fluid pressure within the joint.[15,18,19]

In 2002, Marijnissen and colleagues[20] published a large multicenter prospective study of 57 patients with a mean age of 44 years who underwent ankle distraction and ankle arthroscopy when necessary. Patients were followed on average of 2.8 years. Eleven of the 57 patients were excluded from the study because of short follow-up of less than 1 year and 13 patients withdrew from the study because of recurrent pain and required further treatment. Significant clinical improvement was seen in 38 patients at 1-year follow-up. More importantly, significant functional and clinical improvement was seen compared with the results at 1 year. A randomized study on 17 patients was also performed by the investigators. They evaluated 9 patients with ankle distraction with arthroscopic debridement as necessary compared with 8 patients with arthroscopic debridement alone. The results from the ankle distraction group were similar to their prospective study. In the debridement group, significantly less profound outcomes were observed and 3 of the 8 patients did not reach 1-year follow-up. The failures underwent joint distraction with satisfactory results. In this large multicenter study, significant improvement was observed using joint distraction.

Short-term results of joint distraction have proved to be satisfactory.

Ploegmakers and colleagues[21] performed a multicenter retrospective analysis of 27 patients with posttraumatic osteoarthritis. All patients were treated with Ilizarov ankle distraction. Of the 27 patients, 2 could not be traced and 3 patients incorrectly completed the questionnaire and could not be included in the study. Data was evaluated for these 22 patients with a mean age of 37 years and at least a 7-year follow-up. Six of these patients had remaining persistent pain and went on to arthrodesis. Sixteen patients were evaluated on the basis of pain, function, clinical status, and mobility at a mean 10-year follow-up. Sixteen of the 2-2, or 73%, of patients had significant improvement in all clinical parameters evaluated.

Ankle arthrodiastasis is performed using a circular external ring fixator. Application of a 2-ring block to the tibia is initially achieved. A talar wire is added to prevent distraction of the subtalar joint and is added to the foot plate in addition to the calcaneal wires. The distraction is then performed up to a total of 5 mm at a rate of 0.5 mm 2 times per day. Patients are also allowed to bear weight to tolerance for a recommended treatment duration of at least 3 months.

As with any surgical intervention, ankle arthrodiastasis has complications. The most common complications include soft tissue irritation and superficial infection at pin sites, which can lead to a more serious bone and joint infection. Care should be taken to avoid placing wires intra-articularly because this could cause a septic joint. Improper wire placement can damage neurovascular structures during surgery. Hardware failure can also occur and replacement or removal may be necessary. Overdistraction can lead to ligament tears/damage and fracture. Furthermore, patient noncompliance and psychological issues associated with the frame can become a challenge, therefore the surgeon needs to be prepared for a bailout of the procedure.

Contraindications consist of active infection, vascular impaired limb, poor soft tissue envelope, and significant planal deformities.

The data from multiple studies with large patient populations as well as long-term results show improvement of symptoms and function following ankle joint distraction in patients with severe posttraumatic osteoarthritis. Ankle joint distraction provides a viable joint-sparing treatment of ankle osteoarthritis. Most studies suggest that younger patients benefit more from ankle distraction, although Tellisi and colleagues[15] evaluated age as a predictor of results and showed that patients older than 60 years had more improvement. Even though relief or improvement of symptoms may be temporary, more definitive treatment, such as ankle arthrodesis, can be considered at a later date.

It is the experience of the authors that this provides a reasonable option for patients with end-stage ankle arthritis, in particular for younger patients. The authors suggest that this procedure be reserved for the right patient, and suggest that the patient be fully engaged in preoperative detailed demonstration and explanation of the procedure. In review of the authors experience, we think the condition surrounding joints contributes to the success or failure of the procedure (**Fig. 3**).

ANKLE ARTHRODESIS

Ankle arthrodesis is a well-documented surgical treatment of end-stage ankle arthritis. It has been a preferred treatment of ankle arthritis because of its predictable

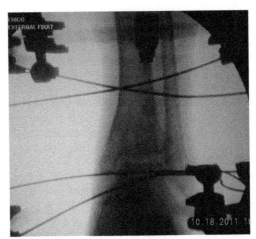

Fig. 3. Arthrodiastasis: an external fixator distracts the ankle joint. Intraoperative image shows 2 smooth wires in the tibia and 2 smooth wires in the talus.

outcomes. In 1879, Albert was the first to described ankle arthrodesis to treat paralytic ankle equinus.[14] More than 30 different techniques to improve the results of the procedure have been described since that time. Ankle arthrodesis is indicated when patients experience persistent pain secondary to the deformity that limits their daily function and after all conservative treatment options have failed.[13,14,22,23] Although still considered the gold standard, ankle arthrodesis for treatment of painful end-stage arthritis, clinicians must be aware of the biomechanical effects on the lower extremity and surrounding joints.

In earlier studies, surgeons experienced high nonunion rates and a higher need for revision surgery. Recent literature reports higher rates of fusion, although variability of fusion rates do exist. Studies report successful union rates of 81% to 99%.[22,24–27] High rates of nonunion have been associated with use of the external compression clamp that was popularized by Charley.[22,26,27] In contrast, in ankle arthrodesis, internal fixation has been associated with higher rates of union.[24,27–30] Morgan and colleagues[28] reviewed 101 ankle joint fusions with an average follow-up for patients of 10 years. An anterolateral surgical approach was used to gain access to the ankle joint and arthrodesis was achieved with screw fixation. A 95% fusion success rate was reported, which can be attributed to their emphasis on preparation of the joint to achieve bone-on-bone contact and use of internal fixation. Zwipp and colleagues[24] reported a fusion rate of 99% in 93 out of 94 patients using a 4-screw technique. Using an anterior fusion plate, Rowan and colleagues[27] achieved a 92% fusion rate in 31 out of 34 patients.

Following ankle arthrodesis, patients notice significant decrease in steps per minute, in addition to decreased stride length, but do not have a significant amount of pain compared with the control group. No significant difference in range of motion in the sagittal plane of the pelvis or the knee joint was seen but fusion of the ankle showed significant decrease in range of motion of the hindfoot and forefoot in all planes (sagittal, transverse, and frontal).[31] Buck and colleagues[32] studied the importance of position of ankle fusion and its affects on patterns of motion of the hindfoot and effect of different ground conditions. The recommended that the optimal position of the ankle joint is neutral flexion, 0° to 5° of valgus of hindfoot angulation and 5° to 10° of external rotation of the foot. A dorsiflexed position is better tolerated than a plantarflexed position of ankle fusion because it decreases sagittal plane motion of the foot and also causes genu recurvatum, producing an abnormal gait that is exaggerated with different ground conditions. Increased extension of the knee is also caused by anterior position of the talus on the tibia and during ambulation uphill. Varus hindfoot position produces a supinated foot type causing locking of the midtarsal joint, whereas arthrodesis in a slight valgus position allows greater motion in the foot. In the stance phase of gait, internal rotation of the foot decreases hindfoot motion and external positioning is indicated to decrease medial collateral ligament stress during toe-off.

Most patients who undergo ankle arthrodesis are satisfied with their results and would go through surgery again in the same circumstances.[25,28,30–33] However, they have long-term functional limitations secondary to pain in adjacent joints.[34] Early postoperative results show no significant changes in adjacent joints, but in one long-term study[35] and another by Coester and colleagues[34] there were significant arthritic changes in adjacent ipsilateral joints compared with the contralateral extremity. Patients had increased osteoarthritic changes in subtalar, talonavicular, and calcaneocuboid joints. In a long-term follow-up study on quality of life by Fuchs and colleagues,[33] 17 patients were followed up for at least for 20 years after ankle arthrodesis. Charnley compression clamps were used in 14 patients as an external fixator for ankle arthrodesis. Only half of the patients had minor restrictions of activities of daily living. Sixteen of the 17 patients were still working and 44% returned to their preinjured occupations, with others performing lighter duties. Similar results were found by Buck and colleagues.[32] Patients had increased physical limitations, emotional disturbance, and pain compared with the age-matched normal population. Significant correlation between functional outcome and radiographic osteoarthritic changes were seen in subtalar joints but not in midtarsal joints. A larger study of 107 subjects was performed by Slobogean and colleagues.[36] Their prospective study evaluated patients with ankle arthrodesis and ankle arthroplasty and their health state values using an SF-36 generic health-related quality of life instrument. The SF-36 uses 11 items to create 6 dimensions (SF-6D), namely physical function, role limitation, social functioning, bodily pain, mental health, and vitality. Patients were evaluated at baseline and at 1 year. They found no statistical difference in results at baseline or 1 year between the ankle arthrodesis or arthroplasty groups. Significant improvement in SF-6D scores were seen between baseline and 1-year follow-up of ankle arthrodesis and ankle arthroplasty groups. At 1-year follow-up, patients' SF-6D results approached age-matched and gender-matched US population norms.

Jung and colleagues[37] evaluated 12 cadaver limbs with an average age of specimen of 68 years (range 52–88 years). A 700-N load was tested on all cadaver specimens. The researchers measured joint contact pressures, peak pressure, and contact area in the talonavicular, subtalar, and calcaneocuboid joints before and after immobilization at neutral ankle axial loading and at tibiopedal dorsiflexion at different angles. Evaluation of different angles was meant to simulate late stance phase of the gait cycle. The results showed that there was significant increase in contact and peak pressures in talonavicular and calcaneocuboid joints between intact and fused ankles at different degrees of dorsiflexion. Comparison of the subtalar joint in intact and fused ankles showed no significant difference in contact or peak pressures but had an increase in contact surface area. Similar results were recorded by Suckel and colleagues[38] in 8 cadaver specimens. Further, an increase in peak pressures were seen at the talonavicular joints. These results suggest that increase in peak pressures at the talonavicular joint may lead to cartilage degeneration and long-term pain along the medial column.

Indications for ankle arthrodesis consist of osteoarthritis, rheumatoid arthritis, septic arthritis, isolated ankle joint Charcot arthropathy, paralytic/neuromuscular conditions, chronic ankle pain, end-stage ankle arthritis, chronic ankle instability, unsuccessful osteochondral defect repair, failed ankle arthroplasty, failed previous ankle arthrodesis, hemophilia, bone tumor, flat top talus, talar avascular necrosis, ankle deformity, and malalignment. Contraindications consist of acute infection and avascular limb.

The goals of an ankle arthrodesis is to reduce pain, improve function, reduce the deformity, provide stability and alignment, and create a plantigrade pain-free foot and ankle. In achieving these goals, the aim is to have the patient return to normal functional activity as much as possible. These activities include returning to a reasonable occupation, independence, and being as ambulatory as possible. Other considerations that need to be taken into account consist of the patient's age, weight, compliance, expectations, other medical conditions, and tobacco use. Because of the development of secondary arthritis, age must be discussed with patients. A young patient who undergoes an ankle arthrodesis may need to have a pantalar arthrodesis many years later. In nonneuropathic patients, this is a procedure the surgeon and patient should try to avoid at all cost.

Many approaches have been described. They consist of anterior, anterior-lateral, medial, lateral, transmalleolar, and posterior. It is the authors experience that the anterior and posterior approach allow the best ease of correction, especially with a frontal plane deformity. Each approach has its own benefit and downside. The posterior approach is favored when there is soft tissue compromise because the soft tissue envelope is thicker and rich in vascularity because of a low-lying flexor hallucis muscle below. Joint preparation can be performed as either curettage, joint resection, burring, or fish scaling. Each of these techniques has its own advantages and disadvantages too. It is the authors' experience that the curettage technique allows the least amount of shortening, provides excellent contour and inherent stability, with excellent bone-to-bone contact, therefore it is the technique of choice of the authors. Fixation options consists of internal fixation and external fixation. The internal fixation for the tibial-talar joint can be a choice of screws, staples, and plates. The authors' first choice is to use large cancellous screws combined with a locking plate and an onlay graft from the fibula as a biologic fixation. The authors highly recommend leaving the fibula intact because this allows patients and the surgeon the option of performing a takedown in the future. This method allows for the possibility of an ankle arthrodesis to be converted to an ankle replacement if needed (**Figs. 4–9**).

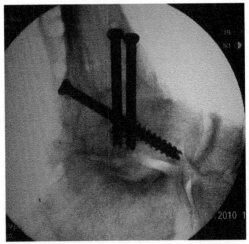

Fig. 4. An intraoperative image showing an ankle fusion fixated with 3 large cancellous screws.

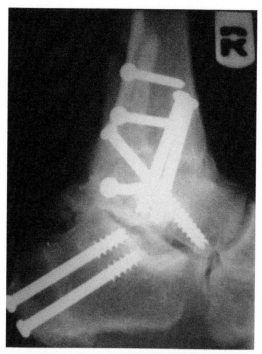

Fig. 5. A postoperative lateral view showing a tibial-talar arthrodesis that is constructed with 3 large cancellous screws at the tibial-talar joint and 3 fibula-tibia screws as a biologic fixation at the tibial-fibula interface.

A variety of complications following ankle arthrodesis have been documented. Neurovascular injury such as nerve damage and arterial/venous laceration sustained during the operation can be avoided with meticulous technique. Careful dissection and a well-planned longitudinal incision can also help minimize the risk to neurovascular complications. Skin complications have been reported 3% to 19% of the time. Most of the issues were superficial skin infections that were treated with oral antibiotics.[25–28] Morgan and colleagues[28] reported 1 deep infection and Rowan and colleagues[27] reported 2 out of 4 deep infections for which intravenous antibiotics were used and debridement preformed.

Rates of delayed union, nonunion, and malunion varied between different studies. Smoking and excessive soft tissue stripping have been associated with nonunion of any fracture or arthrodesis site. This group of patients is at a 4 times greater risk of developing nonunion than those who do not smoke. Nonunion occurs at lower rates when internal hardware has been used for fixation of ankle arthrodesis.[27–30] Malunion following this procedure can have significant effects on patients' gait cycle and can affect surrounding joints secondary to compensation.[32] Other complications consist of secondary arthritis of the subtalar joint and midtarsal joint, avascular necrosis, wound dehiscence, and malalignment. Additional complications such as stress fractures, below-knee amputation, and painful hardware have been reported.

TOTAL ANKLE ARTHROPLASTY

The ankle joint is a complex universal joint that consist of an upper (tibial-talar) and lower (subtalar) ankle joint. The tibial-talar joint is only half of a more complex universal

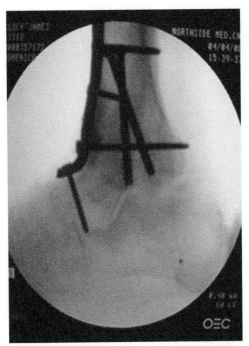

Fig. 6. The use of 2 interfragmentary compression screws coupled with an anterior ankle arthrodesis locking plate.

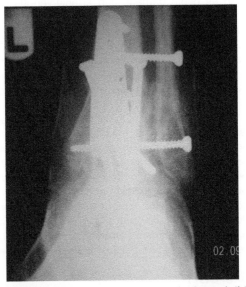

Fig. 7. An anterior-posterior radiograph following a tibial-talar and tibial-fibula arthrodesis using interfragmentary compression screws at the tibial-talar joint, an anterior ankle arthrodesis, and fibula-tibia syndesmosis fusion.

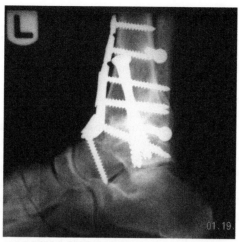

Fig. 8. A lateral radiograph following a tibial-talar and tibial-fibula arthrodesis using inter-fragmentary compression screws at the tibial-talar joint, an anterior ankle arthrodesis, and fibula-tibia syndesmosis fusion.

joint and works together with the other half—the subtalar joint. The problem with a total ankle replacement is that the only part being replaced is the tibial-talar joint. The anatomy of the subtalar joint is complex, therefore it is not replaceable. A normal subtalar joint allows the foot to be flexible, provides stability, and maintains alignment.

Ankle joint replacement works better in patients who are older and have less high-impact activity. Total ankle arthroplasty (TAA) is a viable alternative to ankle arthrodesis for treatment of patients with end-stage ankle arthritis. However, because of poor early results, ankle arthrodesis is considered to be the gold standard for treatment of ankle joint arthritis.[39–43] The initial implants had poor mechanical design, the physicians inserting the ankles had limited experience, therefore the performance of the early generations of ankle implants resulted in a negative stigma. Ankle fusion consequently remains the treatment of choice.

The new generation of ankle implants have better anatomic design, thus are becoming increasingly popular as an alternative to ankle arthrodesis. As a result of

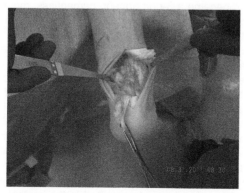

Fig. 9. A posterior approach can be used with a compromised medial, lateral, or anterior soft tissue envelope.

this increasing use of ankle implants, the merits of ankle replacement versus ankle arthrodesis continues to be one of the most debated topics in foot and ankle surgery. Consumers now have access to more information about their health care and, because of this, consumers are researching their options and tending to desire ankle replacement rather than ankle fusion. Patients are also living longer and are more active.

TAA was first performed by Lord and Marrotte in 1970.[10,41,44] The implant design was similar to those used for hip replacements. At a 10-year follow-up, only 7 patients had satisfactory results. First-generation implant design flaws led to a high revision rate. Subsidence and osteolysis was noted with these systems. Loosening of the implant components was seen in constrained designs at their cement-bone interface because normal triplane ankle motion was not addressed. Constrained ankle implant designs provide the greater stability and resistance to wear of polyethylene when surfaces are congruent. Incongruent surfaces in total ankle implants lead to higher stresses on the polyethylene piece, increasing its wear.[10,41,42,44] Because of high failure rates, newer generation implants were developed. They are grouped into 2-component or 3-component designs and as fixed-bearing or mobile-bearing designs.[41,44]

There are currently 5 ankle implants approved by the US Food and Drug Administration (FDA) , although many other systems are used in Europe. Only 1 of the 5 implants is a 3-component design. Agility LP Total Ankle System (DePuy), INBONE Total Ankle (Wright Medical), Salto Talaris Ankle (Tornier), and Eclipse Total Ankle (Integra Life-Sciences) are fixed-bearing, 2-component designs. Even though these implants have 3 pieces, the polyethylene component is fixed to the tibial piece and acts as a 2-component implant. They are considered to be fixed-bearing designs because the polyethylene piece has no independent movement. Scandinavian Total Ankle Replacement (STAR) (SBI) is the only cementless, 3-component, mobile-bearing system that is FDA approved.[39,41,44]

In 1984, Dr Frank Alvine designed the Agility ankle joint implant. Until 2007, it was the only total ankle replacement system that was FDA approved. It requires application of an external fixator to allow distraction of the joint during surgery. Arthrodesis across the syndesmosis is performed to improve stability and to provide support for the tibial component.[39,41,44] The INBONE system is unique. It has an intramedullary alignment system with a multipiece tibial stem. The Salto Talaris ankle implant is a mobile-bearing, 3-component system that is currently used in Europe. It has been redesigned to a 2-component system for use in the United States. In 1978, the STAR was designed as a 2-component, cemented, unconstrained system by Dr Hakon Kofoed. It was not until years later that it became a 3-component, cementless, mobile-bearing system. The STAR design enhances fixation to the tibia through 2 anchorage bars and allows minimal bone resection. The talar component has a longitudinal ridge that stabilizes the polyethylene component during ankle joint motion, and the flat proximal surface allows rotation at the polyethylene and tibial interface.[10,39,41,44]

Proper patient selection is important to achieve successful surgical results, although no absolute criteria have been set.[10,39–42,45] Indications consist of end-stage arthritis from posttraumatic arthritis, primary osteoarthritis, and rheumatoid arthritis. Multiple studies reviewed by Clare and colleagues[40] show that patients 50 years of age and older who underwent TAA had more favorable surgical results than younger patients. Ideal candidates are patients who have adequate bone stock, intact neurovascular status, neutral ankle alignment, intact deltoid ligaments, and are not immunosuppressed.[40–42] When planning TAA, the body weight of a patient is also considered. Obese patients have increased forces transmitted to the implant, making it prone to failure. Other relative contraindications are poor bone stock, immunosuppression, smoking, ankle malalignment, history of septic arthritis, and diabetes. TAA is absolutely contraindicated in patients with high physical demands, poor vascular status, significant neuropathy, infection, neuromuscular deficits, avascular necrosis of the talar body, chronic pain syndrome, and noncompliance.[40–42,46] Ankle malalignment should be avoided to achieve successful ankle joint replacement. Deformities may arise below the ankle joint, at the ankle joint, or above the ankle joint.[46] Flatfoot is the most common deformity located below the ankle joint that contributes to malalignment. The surgeon should address the underlying condition to achieve a tripod effect with the first and fifth metatarsals and a heel in neutral.[40] Deformity arising at the ankle joint may be caused by posttraumatic arthritis or a history of ankle sprains causing a varus ankle joint.[2,46] Patients should also be evaluated for ankle equinus. A Silfverskiold examination is used to assess ankle dorsiflexion with knee bent and extended, with hindfoot in neutral. When decreased ankle dorsiflexion is noted, Achilles tendon lengthening or gastrocnemius recession is then performed according to the results of the Silverskiold test.

Complications following TAA can be attributed to inappropriate patient selection, surgeon experience, and surgeon error.[42] Proper patient selection decreases the risk of complications. Thorough preoperative patient evaluation as well as following clinical guidelines can help achieve a successful surgical outcome.[42,46,47] In addition, outcomes of ankle implants are directly related to the surgeon's experience. Studies show an increase in 5-year survival of ankle implants when a surgeon has performed more than 30 procedures.[42–44] According to a study by Myerson and colleagues,[48] the rates of wound complications decreased from 24% to 8% with increased surgeon experience. A decrease in intraoperative complications including tendon lacerations, nerve laceration, and malleolar fractures has also been seen as a result of accommodation for the steep learning curve.[47,48] According to Mann,[49] complications for this procedure can be divided into 3 groups: low, medium, and high grade, using the Glazebrook classification system. Nine of the 78 ankles (12%) had high-grade complications that included aseptic loosening, deep infection, and implant failure in 4 ankles. Subsidence and postoperative malleolar fracture accounted for 6 patients (7%) with medium-grade complications. Low-grade complications included 6 patients (7%) with superficial skin infection and intraoperative malleolar fractures. Aseptic loosening is associated with pain and, radiographically, a dark halo around the loose component. It is caused by disruption or insufficient bony ingrowth.[42] Deep infection occurred in 3 patients and they were treated with open debridement and 6 weeks of intravenous antibiotics, with no recurrence of infection seen at 9-year follow-up. Osteolysis is lucency seen on radiographs that is typically caused by microscopic debris causing a mediated response or mechanical lysis.[42] Failure of the implants occurred as a result of osteolysis in 2 of the 4 ankles. One ankle implant failed secondary to fracture of the polyethylene piece from forceful axial loading. All 4 ankles were revised and functioning well at 6-year follow-up.[49] Subsidence of the implant may be seen and can be caused by soft bone, overly aggressive bone resection, improper prosthesis placement, sepsis, and an implant that is too small. If this occurs, revision of ankle implant or ankle arthrodesis should be considered.[42] Mann and colleagues[49] noted subsidence in 3 of the patients who had an ankle fusion as a result. Malleolar fractures are associated with surgeon error during the intraoperative period by inappropriate use of a saw blade, which thereby weakens the bone.[10,42]

Failing to address ankle malalignment can cause malleolar fractures during the postoperative period.[42] With superficial skin infection, wound dehiscence ranges vary from 2% to 40% following TAA.[48] Early, conservative local wound care and oral antibiotics can help prevent further complications. According to Saltzman,[50] nerve injury was seen in 20.3% of patients who underwent TAA, compared with 7.6% of patients who had ankle fusion. During surgery, care must be taken to avoid nerve damage to the superficial or deep peroneal nerve. Injury to either nerve is usually a result of laceration or traction.[42] Studies show that medial and lateral gutters of the ankle can be painful after ankle arthroplasty. Spirt and colleagues[51] noted 58 gutter debridements in reoperation of 127 ankles. Eight of the 3-4 ankles had pain in the medial gutter, as reported by Kurup.[52]

Higher revision rates are associated with TAA compared with ankle arthrodesis. Spirt and colleagues[51] noted a 28% revision rate in 306 ankle arthroplasties. A large study performed by SooHoo and colleagues[53] reviewed a total of 4705 ankle fusions and 480 ankle implants. Higher rates of revision surgery were needed: 9% at 1 year and 23% at 5 years in patients who underwent TAA, versus 5% and 11% for ankle fusion. In contrast, Haddad and colleagues,[54] in their review of 1262 patients, found that the rate of revision surgery was lower in patients with ankle implants, at 7% compared with 9% with ankle arthrodesis. When TAA has failed and revision of an implant is impossible, ankle arthrodesis may be the only option before below-the-knee amputation is considered.[13] In a study of 306 ankle arthroplasties, below-knee amputation was performed in 8 patients. Below-knee amputation and deep vein thrombosis are some of the other complications that can occur. In a study by Spirt,[51] amputations were performed because of severe pain in 4 patients and infection in 3 other patients. One of the patients considered below-knee amputation as a surgical option even before undergoing TAA. All patients who underwent below-knee amputation had preoperative hindfoot malalignment.[51]

The authors' experience with ankle replacement surgery has been successful and suggests that it is an acceptable alternative in the treatment of end-stage ankle arthritis when done with protocol-driven indications and appropriate associated conjunctive procedures. The authors think that the key is selecting the right patient, performing a complete evaluation of the extremity, and evaluating a good bone to body size. The patient whose underlying disorder is not corrected before or at the time of implantation is highly susceptible to failure. Patient whose activity levels are altered to meet a lower physical demand and who are conscious of their limitations seem to do the best. The use of an ankle replacement continues to become more predictable when these guidelines are followed.

Because primary osteoarthritis is not common in the ankle joint, the patient population with the highest need of a total ankle is a younger population, usually stemming from posttraumatic arthritis. The ankle replacement surgery is best suited for older patients with degenerative joint disease of the ankle and not involving the subtalar joint, without surrounding soft tissue disorder. However, this patient population is the minority who suffer from end-stage ankle arthritis because pure osteoarthritis in the ankle joint is almost nonexistent. Options for the younger population consist of ongoing physical limitations with pain, amputation, or possible attempt at total ankle replacement. In the younger population who will undergo ankle replacement surgery, it is inevitable that revision and additional surgery will be needed (**Figs. 10–15**).

TOTAL ANKLE ALLOGRAFT TRANSPLANT REPLACEMENT

Fresh bipolar osteochondral allograft of the ankle joint has been sporadically reported in the literature as another alternative to ankle fusion. Allograft transplant replacement uses a fresh graft of the ankle harvested from a cadaver. Similar to total ankle replacement, ankle allograft replacement permits a more normal function. The main advantage of the allograft ankle replacement is the return of some movement in the ankle

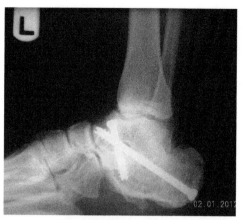

Fig. 10. A preoperative lateral radiograph with secondary ankle joint arthritis and a subtalar joint arthrodesis. A tibial-talar joint arthrodesis coupled with an already subtalar joint fusion most likely leads to further periarticular breakdown. In this case, the foot and ankle surgeon may consider a TAA to prevent further arthrodesis.

with a biologic implant. The potential complications are similar to other operations: the specific concern of the allograft replacement is that the bone and cartilage that is transplanted may not heal, and further arthritis may develop. If this complication occurs with large bony defects, it can be converted to a more traditional total ankle replacement, or even an ankle fusion.

The main advantage of this type of procedure is the potential for replacement of the ankle joint with viable living cartilage cells. The most important aspect of the transplant is the correct sizing to match the ankle. Kadakia and colleagues[55] reported a high failure rate and high revision rate in patients who underwent osteoarticular ankle allograft replacement, which they attributed to high body mass index and a more active

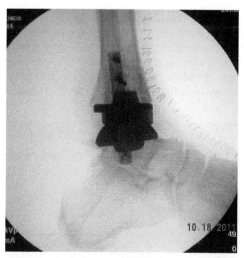

Fig. 11. An intraoperative image of a total ankle replacement using an Agility ankle replacement.

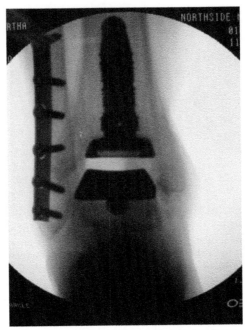

Fig. 12. An intraoperative image of an INBONE total ankle replacement.

patient population. To avoid failure, they suggested that surgeons carefully select patients, that they handle the implants with care, use cutting guides for accuracy, and place the graft early because cartilage is nonviable after 18 days.

Supramalleolar Osteotomy

Supramalleolar osteotomy is a surgical procedure to correct a congenital or acquired deformity of the distal tibia to improve the function of the foot and ankle. This osteotomy is a joint-sparing procedure performed in the juxta-articular region of the tibia. A supramalleolar osteotomy can correct deformities in all planes. Rarely are deformities of the distal tibia managed only by a corrective osteotomy. The frequent existence of accompanying end-stage ankle arthritis is accountable for the clinical symptoms. Indications for a low tibial osteotomy consist of malunited ankle/plafond and distal tibial fractures, congenital deformities, ankle arthritis stemming from the tibial side of the joint, and

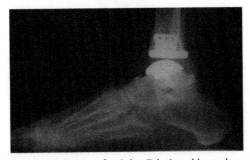

Fig. 13. A postoperative lateral image of a Salto Talaris ankle replacement.

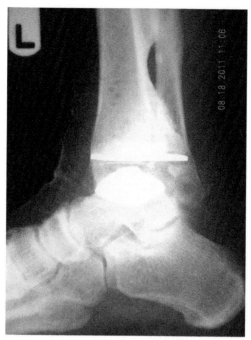

Fig. 14. A postoperative lateral image showing a STAR ankle replacement.

growth plate injuries.[56] Other indications include juxta-articular tibial deformities, mala-ligned arthrodesis, paralytic disorders, and tibial torsion.[57,58] Contraindications consist of impaired neurovascular status, active skin infection, active bone infection, and other comorbidities. Standard anterior-posterior and lateral radiographs of the foot and ankle along with long leg calcaneal axial, rearfoot alignment views of the tibia and fibula, and possibly the knee, can assist in identifying the level of the deformity. The radiographs are used to describe the following characteristics: limb alignment, joint orientation, anatomic axes, mechanical axes, and center of rotation of angulation (CORA).

Normative values for the relations among these various parameters are used to assess deformities. The CORA is the apex of the deformity, consisting of the distal and proximal diaphyseal lines. The distal tibial deformities present with osteoarthritic changes of the ankle joint, or are associated with an ankle fusion malunion. Clinical deformities may or may not be evident, but chronic pain and an increase in pain

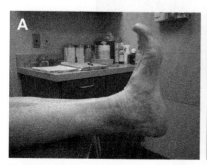
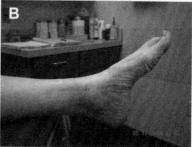

Fig. 15. The amount of (*A*) flexion and (*B*) extension following the implantation of a STAR ankle replacement.

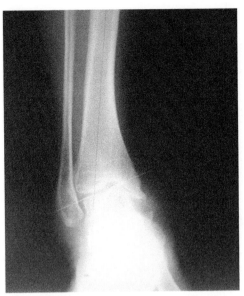

Fig. 16. An anterior view of a patient who has an ankle varus with end-stage ankle arthritis secondary to a physeal arrest. This patient would benefit from a prophylactic tarsal tunnel decompression and a supramalleolar osteotomy.

with usage is common. Because of the natural motion of the subtalar joint, a mild-moderate distal tibial deformity is well tolerated with a rearfoot and midfoot that is supple. In cases with inadequate compensatory motion, the deformity is poorly tolerated. The ability of the foot to compensate for the deformity above the ankle depends on the flexibility of the foot. In scenarios in which a frontal plane deformity such as distal tibia varus or valgus, the forefoot must be able to compensate to remain plantigrade. In scenarios of a stiff hindfoot, there is less capacity for the foot to compensate. Because the naturally occurring subtalar joint motion provides more inversion and less eversion, in scenarios with an unaffected subtalar joint, the hindfoot can compensate for a valgus supramalleolar deformity better than it can compensate for a varus tibial malunion. The soft tissue envelope must be examined well and taken into consideration. An acute correction of the deformity may cause stress on the

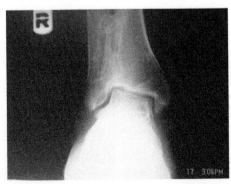

Fig. 17. A patient with an ankle valgus with end-stage ankle joint arthritis secondary to trauma. A supramalleolar osteotomy and a fibular lengthening is needed for realignment.

soft tissues and, in particular, the posterior tibial nerve. A tarsal tunnel syndrome can be caused with an acute varus or procurvatum correction. In patients who present with these conditions, the surgeon should consider a prophylactic tarsal tunnel release.

When performing the osteotomy, the goal is to create the osteotomy as close as possible to the level of the deformity to restore abnormal angles to as close to normal as possible and realign the center of the ankle joint for proper biomechanical function. Performing an osteotomy away from the apex of the deformity corrects the deformity and causes translation. The osteotomy can be a wedge cut, straight cut, or a focal dome osteotomy. Advantages of a focal dome osteotomy consist of a lack of thermal necrosis, minimal periosteal dissection, it can be performed percutaneously, and that it has inherent stability with excellent bone-to-bone contact. The osteotomy accounts for the angular and translational components of a typical opening or closing wedge osteotomy. Focal dome osteotomies minimize the lengthening and shortening of the tibia.[58] Numerous fixation methods have been used to achieve stability at the osteotomy site. Fixation techniques consist of a multitude of internal and external fixation constructs. Contraindications consist of impaired neurovascular status, active skin infections, and active bone infections (**Figs. 16** and **17**).

SUMMARY

End-stage ankle arthritis is a debilitating condition that leads to pain and swelling in the ankle joint, with symptoms aggravated by standing and ambulation. Ankle arthritis commonly results from a history of trauma, or a series of recurrent injuries to the ankle. However, it may develop from other causes such as uneven loading of the ankle joint caused by an alignment deformity or from inflammatory arthritis such as rheumatoid arthritis, gout, or secondary to a serious joint infection. Patients with severe ankle arthritis often have limited ankle motion with an antalgic gait.

Nonoperative treatment is designed to improve function and decrease pain and is based on limiting the amount of loading through the ankle joint, masking the symptoms with antiinflammatory medication and pain medications. Nonoperative care can consist of ankle bracing and rocker-bottom shoe wear.

Operative treatment may be helpful if nonoperative treatment is unsuccessful. These options consist of joint-sparing and joint-destructive procedures. Ankle arthrodesis currently remains the gold standard for advanced ankle arthritis. Although predictable, this procedure has long-term consequences that the surgeon must consider. Available joint-sparing procedures consist of arthrodiastasis, total ankle allograft replacement, supramalleolar osteotomies, and total ankle replacements. Despite promising reports, it has been the authors experience that ankle arthrodiastasis has limitations and realistic expectations are needed regarding long-term results. The authors therefore use this procedure in younger patients who are too young to have an ankle arthroplasty and do not want a fusion. With mixed and limited reports on total ankle allograft replacement, this is a procedure that needs to be assessed more in the years to come. Supramalleolar osteotomies are performed to realign the distal tibia and improve foot and ankle function in those patients who suffer from end-stage ankle joint arthritis and juxta-articular tibial deformity. In the right scenario, this procedure can be powerful and possibly delay additional surgery to the ankle joint.

Newer ankle implants provide patients with decreased pain and improved function. However, these patients must be educated on future physical limitations. Current clinical outcomes of ankle replacement are satisfactory and are more predictable. In terms of function, the ankle replacement is better than an ankle fusion. Ankle replacement preserves motion at the ankle and allows improved function. The motion of the ankle implant also provides a protective function for the remaining joints in the foot, which can develop arthritis because of increased stress of a fused ankle. As more ankle replacements are inserted and more surgeons are performing the procedures, the medical industry will continue to expand, refine, and improve the already successful ankle implants. With increasing supportive medical literature and predictable outcomes, the authors think that implants will continue to be the procedure of choice for selected patients who suffer from end-stage ankle arthritis.

REFERENCES

1. Koh J, Dietz J. Osteoarthritis in other joints (hip, elbow, foot, ankle, toes, wrist) after sports injuries. Clin Sports Med 2005;24:57–70.
2. Valderrabano V, Horisberger M, Russell I, et al. Etiology of ankle osteoarthritis. Clin Orthop Relat Res 2009;467:1800–6.
3. Glazebrook M, Daniels T, Younger A, et al. Comparison of heath-related quality of life between patients with end-stage ankle and hip arthritis. J Bone Joint Surg Am 2008;90:499–505.
4. CDC. Available at: http://www.cdc.gov/chronicdisease/resources/publications/aag/arthritis.htm. Accessed October 20, 2011.
5. Agel J, Coetzee JC, Sangeorzan BJ, et al. Functional limitations of patients with end-stage ankle arthrosis. Foot Ankle Int 2005;26:537–9.
6. Saltzman CL, Salamon MI, Blanchard MG, et al. Epidemiology of ankle arthritis: report of a consecutive series of 639 patients from a tertiary orthopaedic center. Iowa Orthop J 2005;25:44–6.
7. Danies T, Thomas R. Etiology and biomechanics of ankle arthritis. Foot Ankle Clin 2008;13:341–52.
8. Gunther KP, Sturmer T, Sauerland S, et al. Prevalence of generalized osteoarthritis in patients with advanced hip and knee osteoarthritis: the Ulm osteoarthritis study. Ann Rheum Dis 1998;57:717–23.
9. DiDomenico LA, Treadwell JR, Cain LZ. Total ankle arthroplasty in the rheumatoid patient. Clin Podiatr Med Surg 2010;27(2):295–311.
10. Hintermann B, Valderrabano V. Total ankle replacement. Foot Ankle Clin 2003; 8(2):375–405.
11. Cushnaghan J, Dieppe P. Study of 500 patients with limb joint osteoarthritis. I. Analysis by age, sex, and distribution of symptomatic joint sites. Ann Rheum Dis 1991;50: 8–13.
12. Berlet GC, DiDomenico LA, Panchbhavi VK, et al. Roundtable discussion: ankle arthritis. Foot Ankle Spec 2008;1:108–11.
13. Thomas R, Daniels T. Current concepts review: ankle arthritis. J Bone Joint Surg Am 2003;85:923–36.
14. Scranton PE. An overview of ankle arthrodesis. Clin Orthop Relat Res 1991;268: 96–101.
15. Tellisi N, Fragomen AT, Kleinman D, et al. Joint preservation of the osteoarthritic ankle using distraction arthroplasty. Foot Ankle Int 2009;30(4):318–25.
16. Chiodo CP, McGarvey W. Joint distraction for the treatment of ankle osteoarthritis. Foot Ankle Clin North Am 2004;9:541–53.
17. van Volburg AA, van Roenmund PM, Marijnissen AC, et al. Joint distraction in treatment of osteoarthritis: a two-year follow-up of the ankle. Osteoarthr Cartil 1999;7(5):474–9.
18. Paley D, Lamm BM. Ankle joint distraction. Foot Ankle Clin North Am 2005;10: 685–98.

19. Kluesner AJ, Wukich DK. Ankle arthrodiastasis. Clin Podiatr Med Surg 2009; 26(2):227–44.
20. Marijnissen AC, van Roermund PM, van Melkebeek J, et al. Clinical benefit of joint distraction in the treatment of severe osteoarthritis of the ankle. Arthritis Rheum 2002;46(11):2893–902.
21. Ploegmakers JJW, van Roermund PM, van Melkebeek J, et al. Prolonged clinical benefit from joint distraction in the treatment of ankle osteoarthritis. J Osteoarthr Cartil 2005;13:582–8.
22. Abidi NA, Gruen GS, Conti SF. Ankle arthrodesis: indications and techniques. J Am Acad Orthop Surg 2000;8(3):200–9.
23. Coughlin MJ, Mann RA, Saltzman CL. Ankle arthritis. Surg Foot Ankle 2007;923–84.
24. Zwipp H, Rammelt S, Endres T, et al. High union rates and function scores at midterm followup with ankle arthrodesis using a four screw technique. Clin Orthop Relat Res 2010;468:958–68.
25. Abdo RV, Wasilewski SA. Ankle arthrodesis: a long-term study. Foot Ankle 1992; 13:307–12.
26. Lynch AF, Bourne RB, Rorabeck CH. The long-term results of ankle arthrodesis. J Bone Joint Surg Am 1988;70:113–7.
27. Rowan R, Davey KJ. Ankle arthrodesis using an anterior AO T plate. J Bone Joint Surg Br 1999;81:113–6.
28. Morgan CD, Henke JA, Bailey RW, et al. Long-term results of tibiotalar arthrodesis. J Bone Joint Surg Am 1985;67:546–9.
29. Dent CM, Patel M, Fairclough JA. Arthroscopic ankle arthrodesis. J Bone Joint Surg Br 1993;75:830–2.
30. Winson IG, Robinson DE, Allen PE. Arthroscopic ankle arthrodesis. J Bone Joint Surg Br 2005;87:343–7.
31. Thomas R, Daniels TR, Parker K. Gait analysis and functional outcomes following ankle arthrodesis for isolated ankle arthritis. J Bone Joint Surg 2006;88(3): 526–35.
32. Buck P, Morrey BF, Chao EY. The optimum position of arthrodesis of the ankle: a gait study of the knee and ankle. J Bone Joint Surg 1987;69(7):1052–62.
33. Fuchs S, Sandmann C, Skwara A, et al. Quality of life 20 years after arthrodesis of the ankle. A study of adjacent joints. J Bone Joint Surg Br 2003;85(7):994–8.
34. Coester LM, Saltzman CL, Leupold J, et al. Long-term results following ankle arthrodesis for post-traumatic arthritis. J Bone Joint Surg Am 2001;83:219–28.
35. Saltzman CL, Kadoko RG, Suh JS. Treatment of isolated ankle osteoarthritis with arthrodesis or the total ankle replacement: a comparison of comparison of early outcomes. Clin Orthop Surg 2010;2:1–7.
36. Slobogean GP, Younger A, Apostly KL, et al. Preference-based quality of life of end-stage ankle arthritis treated with arthroplasty or arthrodesis. Foot Ankle Int 2010;31(7):563–6.
37. Jung HG, Parks BG, Nguyen A, et al. Effect of tibiotalar joint arthrodesis on adjacent tarsal joint pressure in a cadaver model. Foot Ankle Int 2007;28:103–108l.
38. Suckel A, Muller O, Herberts T, et al. Changes in Chopart joint load following tibiotalar arthrodesis: in vitro analysis of 8 cadaver specimens in a dynamic model. BMC Musculoskelet Disord 2007;8:80.
39. Mendicino RW, Catanzariti AR, Peterson KS. Emerging insights with ankle implants arthroplasty. Podiatry Today 2011;24:32–8.
40. Clare MP, Sanders RW. Preoperative consideration in ankle replacement surgery. Foot Ankle Clin 2002;7:709–20.

41. DiDomenico LA, Anania MC. Total ankle replacements: an overview. Clin Podiatr Med Surg 2011;28:727–44.
42. Steck JK, Anderson JB. Total ankle arthroplasty: indication and avoiding complications. Clin Podiatr Med Surg 2009;26:303–24.
43. Dyrby C, Chou LB, Andriacchi TP, et al. Functional evaluation of the Scandinavian Total Ankle Replacement. Foot Ankle Int 2004;25:377–81.
44. Gougoulias NE, Khanna A, Maffulli N. History and evolution in total ankle arthroplasty. Br Med Bull 2009;89:111–51.
45. DiDomenico LA, Camasta CA. Is total ankle replacement more effective than ankle arthrodesis? Podiatry Today 2010;23:50–8.
46. Greisberg J, Hansen ST Jr. Ankle replacement: management of associated deformities. Foot Ankle Clin 2002;7:721–36.
47. Conti SF, Wong YS. Complication of total ankle replacement. Not Found In Database 2001;391:105–14.
48. Myerson MS, Mroczek K. Perioperative complications of total ankle arthroplasty. Foot Ankle Int 2003;24:17–21.
49. Mann JA, Mann RA, Horton E. STAR ankle: long-term results. Foot Ankle Int 2011; 32:473–84.
50. Saltzman CL, Mann RA, Ahrens JE, et al. Prospective controlled trail of STAR total ankle replacement versus ankle fusion: initial results. Foot Ankle Int 2009;30: 579–93.
51. Spirt AA, Assal M, Hansen ST. Complications and failure after total ankle arthroplasty. J Bone Joint Surg Am 2004;86:1172–8.
52. Kurup HV, Taylor GR. Medial impingement after ankle replacement. Int Orthop 2008;32:243–6.
53. SooHoo NF, Zingmond DS, Ko CY. Comparison of reoperation rates following ankle arthrodesis and total ankle arthroplasty. J Bone Joint Surg Am 2007;89: 2143–9.
54. Haddad SL, Coetzee JC, Estok R, et al. Intermediate and long-term outcomes of total ankle arthroplasty and ankle arthrodesis: a systematic review of the literature. J Bone Joint Surg Am 2007;89:1899–905.
55. Kadakia AJ, Jeng C, Myerson M, et al. Osteoarticular ankle allograft replacement. Presented at the American Orthopaedic Foot and Ankle Society 22nd Annual Summer Meeting. La Jolla (CA), July 14–16, 2006.
56. Best A, Daniels TR. Supramalleolar tibial osteotomy secured with the Puddu plate. Foot Ankle Orthop 2006;29(6):537.
57. Mangone PG. Distal tibial osteotomies for the treatment of foot and ankle disorders. Foot Ankle Clin 2001;6:583.
58. Paley D, Herzenberg JE, Tetsworth K, et al. Deformity planning for the frontal plane corrective osteotomies. Orthop Clin North Am 1994;25:425.

Gastrocnemius Recession or Tendo-Achilles Lengthening for Equinus Deformity in the Diabetic Foot?

Robert M. Greenhagen, DPM[a],*, Adam R. Johnson, DPM[b],
Nicholas J. Bevilacqua, DPM[c]

KEYWORDS

- Diabetes mellitus • Equinus • Achilles • Gastrocnemius recession
- Tendo-Achilles lengthening • Limited joint mobility syndrome

KEY POINTS

- Ankle equinus should always be considered as a contributing factor to the underlying cause of a foot deformity or a plantar foot ulceration.
- Differentiation between the need for a gastrocnemius recession and the need for a TAL is based on the degree of the deformity and the cause of the equinus.

 Video of open evaluation of Hoke's triple hemisection accompanies this article at http://www.podiatric.theclinics.com/.

INTRODUCTION

The Achilles tendon is made up of a confluence of tendinous contributions from the gastrocnemius and soleus muscles. This complex is known as the triceps surae. The gastrocnemius muscle is composed of a medial and lateral head, originates on the posterior aspect of the femoral condyle, and courses distally to span 3 joints (knee, ankle, and subtalar joint). The soleus muscle originates from the posterior aspect of the tibia and fibula below the knee and spans across the ankle and subtalar joint. The combined aponeuroses of the gastrocnemius and soleus converge to form the Achilles tendon.

Ankle equinus is a pathologic limitation of ankle joint range of motion caused by a contracted Achilles-gastrocnemius-soleus complex. Researchers have disagreed about the minimum range of motion at the ankle joint required for normal ambulation; however,

[a] Private Practice, Foot and Ankle Center of Nebraska, Omaha, NE, USA; [b] Department of Surgery, Hennepin County Medical Center, Minneapolis, MN, USA; [c] North Jersey Orthopaedic Specialists, PA, Teaneck, NJ, USA
* Corresponding author.
E-mail address: robert.m.greenhagen@dmu.edu

Clin Podiatr Med Surg 29 (2012) 413–424
doi:10.1016/j.cpm.2012.04.005   **podiatric.theclinics.com**
0891-8422/12/$ – see front matter © 2012 Elsevier Inc. All rights reserved.

most agree that at least 10° of dorsiflexion at the ankle is required for normal ambulation. Limited range of motion at the ankle joint is a significant causative factor in the development of abnormal foot function. Ankle equinus (<10° of dorsiflexion) may be the primary pathologic factor in conditions such as clubfoot or neuromuscular diseases or may serve as a causative factor of a disorder that presents in the foot, such as hallux abductovalgus, adult and pediatric flatfoot, Achilles tendinopathy, plantar fasciitis, diabetic foot ulceration, and Charcot neuroarthropathy.[1–3] Ankle equinus may also occur after certain partial foot amputations and may become a causative factor in recurrent ulcerations after certain foot amputations. Treatment of equinus varies and depends on the cause, severity, medical comorbidities, and surgeon preference. Currently, there is no gold standard for the treatment of equinus and some controversy exists as to which method is preferred. This article reviews the basics of equinus and compares the most commonly performed procedures, gastrocnemius recession, tendo-Achilles lengthening (TAL), and Achilles tenotomy.

ANKLE EQUINUS AND THE DIABETIC FOOT

The Centers for Disease Control and Prevention estimated in 2010 that 25.8 million Americans are affected by diabetes[4] and another 79 million are affected by prediabetes. The diabetes epidemic in the United States continues to tax the health care system. It is estimated that up to 25% of people with diabetes mellitus suffer an ulceration within their lifetimes.[5] Therefore, identifying potentially modifiable risk factors for ulceration is key to amputation prevention. One such modifiable risk that may contribute to the formation of ulceration is increased plantar forefoot pressures. Veves and colleagues[6] found that a plantar ulcer occurred in 35% of diabetic patients with high plantar foot pressures, but occurred in none with normal pressures. Increased plantar pressure has been shown to occur early in the onset of diabetes. Boulton and colleagues[7] showed abnormalities in foot pressure occurring early with sensory neuropathy, and this may precede clinical abnormalities. The most important risk factor in the pathogenesis of diabetic foot ulceration is the loss of sensory awareness, which occurs in 60% to 70% of those with diabetes, and therefore high plantar pressure alone is not the cause of ulceration, but rather a casual effect. Frykberg and colleagues[8] found that persons with diabetes have a higher prevalence of ankle equinus as compared to non diabetic persons (37.2% vs 15.3%). The researchers also uncovered a significant association between equines and ulceration.[8]

There are many contributing factors that may lead to increased plantar foot pressures. Some are obvious deformities (ie, bunions and hammertoes); however, a potentially major contributing factor that is often not recognized is limited joint mobility syndrome (LJMS).[9] This syndrome is a wide spectrum of disorders and includes reduced range of motion and tissue elasticity, and muscular imbalance. Ankle equinus is part of this spectrum.

EQUINUS AS A SOURCE OF HIGH PLANTAR FOOT PRESSURES

The reported overall prevalence of equinus in the diabetic population is 10.3%, however, recently Frykberg and colleagues,[8] reported a prevalence of 37.2% in persons with diabetes. Using electron microscopy, Grant and colleagues[10] found structural changes in the Achilles tendons of patients with diabetes, characterized by increased density of collagen fibrils, decreased fibrillar diameter, abnormal fibril morphology, and frequent foci of collagenous fiber disorganization. These fine morphologic changes may be the result of nonenzymatic glycosylation, which, as a result, stiffens the Achilles tendon. As the Achilles loses its flexibility, the foot loses its ability to adequately dorsiflex during gait, creating a longer lever arm and placing abnormal forces on the midfoot.[11] Decreased ankle dorsiflexion results in shifts in distribution of plantar pressures with peak pressures increased under the forefoot.[11]

Patients with equinus have significantly higher peak plantar pressures than those without the deformity and are at nearly 3 times greater risk for presenting with increased plantar pressures.[12] Simulated Achilles tendon contracture increases the severity of arch depression and forefoot abduction.[13] Caselli and colleagues[14] showed an increase in forefoot-to-rearfoot pressure with increasing degrees of neuropathy. This finding lends further evidence for the concept that equinus is a progressive deformity and becomes more severe in the later stages of peripheral neuropathy, thereby playing an important role in the cause of diabetic foot ulceration.

LJMS involves more than just an equinus deformity. Orendruff and colleagues[15] showed that the relationship between equinus and peak forefoot pressure was significant but, by itself, has only a limited role in causing high forefoot pressure. The soft tissue imbalance that occurs in LJMS is also a major factor in increasing plantar pressures. Abboud and colleagues[16] found abnormalities in the tibialis anterior muscle function during the gait cycle in subjects with diabetic peripheral neuropathy. This condition resulted in a prolonged flattening of the foot and a significant increase in plantar pressures.[16] Therefore, understanding the relationship and balancing of the dorsiflexory and plantarflexory muscle groups is important when addressing increased plantar pressure.

Attention must also be given to the balance of forces in the foot after certain partial foot amputations. An Achilles tendon lengthening or a gastrocnemius recession should be performed in conjunction with partial foot amputations at, or proximal to, a transmetatarsal amputation.

PROCEDURE SELECTION

When considering surgical correction of equinus, several factors must be considered during procedure selection. Distinguishing which portion of the triceps surae complex is contracted may assist in determining which procedure will be most effective. Traditionally, the Silfverskiold test (the amount of dorsiflexion is evaluated with the knee straight and bent) has been used as a major decision maker in surgical planning, but this assumption may be flawed. Schweinberger and Roukis[17] suggested that there is no clinically significant difference between an isolated gastrocnemius equinus and a gastrocnemius-soleus equinus because the timing of passive ankle joint dorsiflexion in the gait cycle only occurs with the knee in an extended position until the heel comes off the ground during toe-off. Aronow and colleagues[18] performed a mechanical loading study using 10 fresh frozen cadaveric legs that were loaded with 35.8 kg (79 lb) of plantar force through the isolated gastrocnemius, isolated soleus, or combined gastrocnemius-soleus muscles and found similar redistribution of plantar force from the rearfoot to the midfoot and forefoot in each of the 3 muscle sets tested.

Kay and colleagues[19] performed a retrospective review of 54 ambulatory children with fixed ankle equinus treated with either TAL or gastrocnemius recession. Their study garnered information for procedure selection to help improve future outcomes. The gait laboratory was used to identify patients who would benefit from a procedure to correct ankle equinus; however, procedure selection was not made from this information. Procedure selection was based on static examination of dorsiflexion at the ankle with the knee flexed. The gastrocnemius recession was performed in patients who could dorsiflex to neutral and beyond, whereas the TAL was reserved for patients who were unable to achieve dorsiflexion to neutral. Using this test to determine procedure selection produced an end result with no significant difference in postoperative dorsiflexion, whereas after surgery there was significance.

The surgeon must assess ankle equinus when addressing complex foot and ankle deformities. Addressing the equinus deformity is often necessary when performing a midfoot arthrodesis to align the foot and may serve to unload stress on the midfoot. For hindfoot and ankle fusion procedures, it is imperative to check ankle range of motion and consider lengthening because a lengthening may be required to reposition the hindfoot anatomically.

Several factors should be considered when selecting the proper surgical procedure. Three surgical options exist, including gastrocnemius recession, TAL, and Achilles tenotomy. Each option carries its own risks and benefits, and performing the appropriate procedure enhances the outcome (**Table 1**).

GASTROCNEMIUS RECESSION

Vulpius and Stoffel[20] introduced the gastrocnemius recession in 1913, transecting the gastrocnemius aponeurosis with a chevron cut and incising the deep fibers of the soleus. Several surgical variations have been described since. Silfveskiold released the gastrocnemius from its origin on the femoral condyles and repositioned the muscle below the knee.[21] Strayer[22] performed a transverse sectioning of the gastrocnemius aponeurosis where it attached to the underlying soleus aponeurosis. Baker[23] modified the Vulpius procedure and described a tongue-and-groove recession. Lamm and colleagues[24] describe a technique similar to Vulpius, but modified the technique by making a single transverse cut, rather than a single cut or multiple chevron cuts. Endoscopic procedures have emerged as an alternative to the open technique (**Fig. 1**).[25,26]

Surgeons have also targeted the gastrocnemius aponeurosis of the muscular bound portion. Baumann described multiple transections for cases of cerebral palsy (CP).[27] Blitz and Rush[28] performed a single transection of this muscular bound aponeurosis through a small medial incision, and titled the procedure the gastrocnemius intramuscular aponeurotic recession (GIAR). Based on cadaver study, Blitz and Eliot[29,30] further modified the aponeurotic transection to mirror the angle of the underlying gastrocnemius musculature.

Hamilton and colleagues[31] were the first to report the use of a gastrocnemius recession for the management of diabetic foot ulcer. The procedure was used in combination with more traditional procedures, such as a peroneus longus to brevis transfer, and resection of the second to fifth metatarsal heads. This comprehensive approach led to a 100% healing rate of plantar foot ulceration. Dayer and Assal[32] reported a 96% healing rate with the use of a Strayer gastrocnemius recession, performed in conjunction with a Jones tenosuspension, a flexor hallucis longus transfer from the distal phalanx to the proximal phalanx, and a peroneus longus to brevis transfer. Recently, Greenhagen and colleagues[33] were the first to report the use of an isolated gastrocnemius recession to address a neuropathic forefoot ulceration.

The gastrocnemius recession is indicated for mild to moderate ankle equinus and has several advantages compared with the more commonly performed TAL. First, by lengthening only the gastrocnemius and leaving the soleus intact, the procedure offers a more controlled lengthening, thereby decreasing the risk of overlengthening and rupture of the Achilles tendon.[11,18,33] Second, the gastrocnemius recession maintains plantarflexory strength by preserving the underlying soleus muscle and preserves the integrity of the Achilles tendon near its insertion onto the calcaneus.[34] This procedure spares a potentially pathologic tendon, because there may be a preexisting Achilles tendinopathy present.[35,36] The consequence of further weakening a diseased tendon could exacerbate the degradation and lead to rupture. Third, the surgical site for the gastrocnemius recession surgical site has the advantage of increased vascularity to both the tendon and the skin compared with that of the TAL. Naito and Ogata[37] showed

Table 1
Outline of procedure selection

Procedure	Indications	Benefits	Risk	Recommendation[a]
Gastrocnemius recession	Mild to moderate equinus Insensate calcaneus Inability to remain non–weight bearing History of Achilles tendinopathy	Control lengthening Decrease risk of calcaneal gait Decrease risk of Achilles rupture Decrease risk of nonhealing incision	Inadequate lengthening Recurrent ulceration	Level C
Tendo-Achilles lengthening	Moderate to severe equinus Spastic equinus Recurrent equinus Ankle or TTC fusion Inability to remain non–weight bearing History of Achilles tendinopathy	Moderate correction Ease of procedure	Overlengthening Achilles rupture Calcaneal gait/ulceration	Level A
Achilles tenotomy	Recurrent equinus Severe equinus Spastic equinus Ankle or TTC fusion Capable of non–weight bearing	Significant correction Low risk of equinus recurrence	Overlengthening Calcaneal gait/ulceration	Level C

Abbreviation: TTC, tibiotalocalcaneal fusion.
[a] Based on the US Preventive Services Task Force recommendation categories.

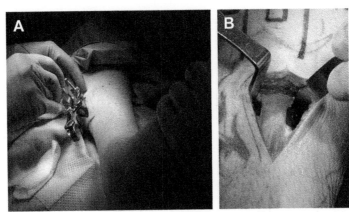

Fig. 1. (*A*) A mini–open gastrocnemius recession performed using a pediatric speculum. (*B*) The use of an open McGlamry gastrocnemius recession for the treatment of equinus.

that 65% of the blood supply to the tendon arises from the musculotendinous junction and the osteotendinous insertional zone. The risk of inadequate or compromised vascular supply increases with distance farther distal from the surgical site on the lower extremity.

In cases of CP, the gastrocnemius recession has been shown to improve calf spasticity, whereas TAL has not.[19] Also of interest in patients with CP, although both TAL and gastrocnemius recession increase push-off power after surgery, only the gastrocnemius recession group has been shown to be significant.[19]

The advantage of the gastrocnemius recession (controlled, limited lengthening) is also potentially a disadvantage. Consequently, the achieved lengthening may be inadequate to restore ankle motion to the proper level. In addition, the recurrence rate of equinus is 3 times that of the TAL, and the gastrocnemius recession carries a 16% recurrence rate of late plantar forefoot reulceration, which may require a repeat procedure.[11] Rush and colleagues[34] evaluated the morbidity associated with the open gastrocnemius recession and found an overall complication rate of 6% after performing 150 procedures. Complications included scar tissue formation, nerve-related disorders including complex regional pain syndrome, and wound dehiscence with and without cellulitis. They noted that failure to repair the paratenon at closure resulted in a poorer outcome for scaring and induration after surgery, and therefore recommended a layered closure with the procedure. Their reported incidence of nerve-related problems in performing open procedures was favorable compared with those found in performing the procedure endoscopically (7%).[25]

TAL

The next option is the TAL. This option is indicated when there is a combined gastrocnemius-soleus complex contracture resulting in moderate to severe equinus deformity. The lengthening may be performed through an open incision, but is often performed through percutaneous incisions to minimize wound complications. This technique is advantageous in patients who have peripheral arterial disease. Yosipovitch and Sheskin[38] were the first to report the use of Achilles tendon lengthening to decrease forefoot pressure as a treatment of forefoot ulcerations in leprosy (**Fig. 2**).

Mueller and colleagues[2] conducted a randomized control trial comparing the combined treatment of total contact cast (TCC) and percutaneous TAL with a TCC

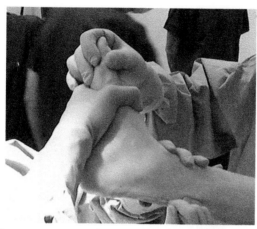

Fig. 2. The use of the percutaneous Hoke triple hemisection as an adjunctive reconstructive procedure.

alone. Initial healing rates were similar in both groups (88% in the group receiving the TCC alone, and 100% in the TAL and TCC group). However, significant difference was noted when comparing the ulcer recurrence rates after 2 years (81% ulcer recurrence rate in the group treated with a TCC alone compared with 38% in those treated with TCC and TAL). This study shows the importance of addressing the underlying equines deformity to augment healing and to reduce the risk of ulcer recurrence.

Armstrong and colleagues[39] studied forefoot pressures via electronic force plate before and after TAL. Mean forefoot pressure decreased from 86 ($\pm$9.4) N/cm^2 to 63 ($\pm$13.2) N/cm^2. Furthermore, mean dorsiflexion of the ankle joint increased from 0° ($\pm$3.1°) to 9° ($\pm$2°) at 8 weeks after surgery. Salsich and colleagues[40] also found that the TAL resulted in an increase in ankle dorsiflexion. More importantly, they showed a temporary reduction in concentric plantarflexor peak torque and passive torque at 0° of dorsiflexion. Therefore, TAL addresses the muscle imbalance between the active dorsiflexory and plantarflexory muscle groups.

Risks are associated with the TAL, such as overlengthening, tendon rupture, and loss of plantarflexory muscle strength. The amount of lengthening is not easily controlled and overlengthening can result in a calcaneal gait and, in patients with an insensate heal, this can result in ulceration.[41,42] The resultant heel ulceration is difficult to heal and may require a sophisticated flap to achieve closure; if not responsive, this may result in a below-knee amputation (**Fig. 3**). Mohsen Allam[43] found calcaneal gait and acute heel ulceration in 16.7% of patients treated with a percutaneous TAL. The risk of a late heel ulcer is 6.7%, 13.3%, and 20% after 6, 12, and 24 months after surgery among TAL cases, and this complication was correlated with excessive ankle dorsiflexion caused by Achilles tendon overlengthening. On average, heel ulceration costs 1.5 times more than metatarsal ulceration; limb salvage of the heel is 2 to 3 times less likely than metatarsal salvage.[44] Caution is advised in patients with complete anesthesia of the heel (Video 1).[45]

Most TAL procedures occur at what Lagergren and Lindholm[46] describe as the watershed area (2–6 cm from the insertion) and therefore tendon rupture may occur (**Fig. 4**). The final risk is postoperative dysfunction and weakness. Stauff and colleagues[47] found that, after a TAL, 80% of patients reported some degree of persistent stiffness and 38% of patients reported postoperative weakness.

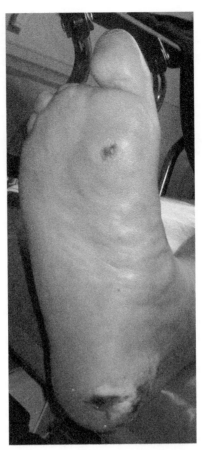

Fig. 3. Heel ulceration secondary to Achilles overlengthening. The patient underwent a percutaneous tendo-Achilles lengthening for the treatment of a forefoot ulceration.

In stance, the soleus muscle is active and important for balance and, as Lamm and colleagues[24] point out, a TAL decreases the strength of the soleus muscle and thereby may impair balance. This finding becomes especially important in people with diabetes and neuropathy, who often have diminished proprioception and, therefore, postural imbalance.

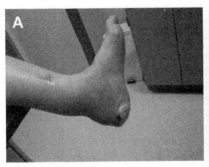
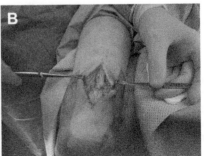

Fig. 4. (*A*) A subsequent heel ulceration can occur and (*B*) rupture of the Achilles tendon can occur after TAL.

ACHILLES TENOTOMY

The final option is an Achilles tenotomy, which offers the most aggressive and definitive option and may be considered in severe equines. Achilles tenotomy is most often used for the treatment of clubfoot or CP contractures. In the diabetic foot, Achilles tenotomy is reserved for severe equinus deformity and may be considered and performed as an adjunctive procedure in conjunction with a Charcot reconstruction, ankle arthrodesis, or a tibiotalocalcaneal arthrodesis. In 1938, Hogden and Frantz[48] reviewed the current opinions of Achilles tenotomy. They noted that TAL is often inadequate for correction of severe equinus and that the procedure is simple and effective. However, after poor results within their clinic and reviewing current opinions of other orthopedic surgeons, they abandoned the use of the Achilles tenotomy. Outside of selected populations, limited data exist to evaluate the use of Achilles tenotomy.

Significant correction can be obtained with a tenotomy. Dogan and colleagues[49] found an average of 20° improvement in ankle dorsiflexion after Achilles tenotomy. Animal studies have shown similar healing and strength in rat tendons after TAL and Achilles tenotomy.[50] As expected, Achilles tenotomy has significant risk of calcaneal gait. Most subjects who undergo tenotomy are not ambulatory, because of age or comorbidities, so the incidence of calcaneal gait is unknown. El-Hawary and colleagues[51] found that 10% (8/79) of subjects showed a calcaneal gait after treatment with the Ponseti method. Other serious risks associated with a percutaneous tenotomy include risk of serious bleeding,[52] pseudoaneurysm,[53] knee hyperextension,[51] and equinus gait.[51]

SUMMARY

Ankle equinus should always be considered as a contributing factor to the underlying cause of a foot deformity or a plantar foot ulceration. Ankle equinus may be the primary pathologic factor or may be a contributing factor in a multifactorial condition. Identifying and addressing an underlying equinus deformity is essential for optimal outcome when dealing with complex foot deformities and diabetic foot ulcerations.

Differentiation between the need for a gastrocnemius recession and the need for a TAL is based on the degree of the deformity and the cause of the equinus.[24] In general, when managing an equinus deformity in the diabetic foot, the authors' preferred approach favors the gastrocnemius recession. In most cases of ankle equinus in this population, a gastrocnemius recession appropriately addresses the deformity while maintaining plantarflexory muscle strength and preserving function. The gastrocnemius recession maintains muscle strength and is preferred to a TAL, which, if overlengthened, causes maximum loss of strength. Although failure of a TAL is uncommon, complications from a TAL may result in more deleterious consequences than the patient's initial presenting problem.

However, in severe equinus deformity, a TAL may be required to obtain the desired length for adequate correction. A TAL may also be required to facilitate ankle dorsiflexion to reposition the hindfoot anatomically in tibiotalar and tibiotalocalcaneal fusions. A percutaneous approach is often used in this high-risk patient population because there is often a component of peripheral arterial disease present. The authors rarely use an Achilles tenotomy, and consider it only in the most severe deformities and in conjunction with an ankle fusion or a tibiotalocalcaneal fusion.

Addressing an equinus deformity may be difficult. It is important to have a sound understanding of the available procedures and appreciate the advantages and disadvantages each procedure offers.

SUPPLEMENTARY DATA

Supplementary data related to this article can be found online at doi:10.1016/j.cpm. 2012.04.005.

REFERENCES

1. Mann RA, Coughlin MJ. Hallux valgus—etiology, anatomy, treatment and surgical considerations. Clin Orthop Relat Res 1981;(157):31–41.
2. Mueller MJ, Sinacore DR, Hastings MK, et al. Effect of Achilles tendon lengthening on neuropathic plantar ulcers. A randomized clinical trial. J Bone Joint Surg Am 2003;85(8):1436–45.
3. Patel A, DiGiovanni B. Association between plantar fasciitis and isolated contracture of the gastrocnemius. Foot Ankle Int 2011;32(1):5–8.
4. Center for Disease Control and Prevention. National diabetes fact sheet: national estimates and general information on diabetes and prediabetes in the United States, 2011. Atlanta (GA): US Department of Health and Human Services, Center for Disease Control and Prevention; 2011.
5. Singh N, Armstrong DG, Lipsky BA. Preventing foot ulcers in patients with diabetes. JAMA 2005;293(2):217–28.
6. Veves A, Murray HJ, Young MJ, et al. The risk of foot ulceration in diabetic patients with high foot pressure: a prospective study. Diabetologia 1992;35(7):660–3.
7. Boulton AJ, Betts RP, Franks CI, et al. Abnormalities of foot pressure in early diabetic neuropathy. Diabet Med 1987;4(3):225–8.
8. Frykberg RG, Bowen J, Hall J, et al. J Am Podiatr Med Assoc 2012;102(2):84–8.
9. Zimny S, Schatz H, Pfohl M. The role of limited joint mobility in diabetic patients with an at-risk foot. Diabetes Care 2004;27(4):942–6.
10. Grant WP, Sullivan R, Sonenshine DE, et al. Electron microscopic investigation of the effects of diabetes mellitus on the Achilles tendon. J Foot Ankle Surg 1997; 36(4):272–8 [discussion: 330].
11. Nishimoto GS, Attinger CE, Cooper PS. Lengthening the Achilles tendon for the treatment of diabetic plantar forefoot ulceration. Surg Clin North Am 2003; 83(3):707–26.
12. Lavery LA, Armstrong DG, Boulton AJ. Ankle equinus deformity and its relationship to high plantar pressure in a large population with diabetes mellitus. J Am Podiatr Med Assoc 2002;92(9):479–82.
13. Blackman AJ, Blevins JJ, Sangeorzan BJ, et al. Cadaveric flatfoot model: ligament attenuation and Achilles tendon overpull. J Orthop Res 2009;27(12):1547–54.
14. Caselli A, Pham H, Giurini JM, et al. The forefoot-to-rearfoot plantar pressure ratio is increased in severe diabetic neuropathy and can predict foot ulceration. Diabetes Care 2002;25(6):1066–71.
15. Orendurff MS, Rohr ES, Sangeorzan BJ, et al. An equinus deformity of the ankle accounts for only a small amount of the increased forefoot plantar pressure in patients with diabetes. J Bone Joint Surg 2006;88(1):65–8.
16. Abboud RJ, Rowley DI, Newton RW. Lower limb muscle dysfunction may contribute to foot ulceration in diabetic patients. Clin Biomech (Bristol, Avon) 2000;15(1):37–45.
17. Schweinberger MH, Roukis TS. Surgical correction of soft-tissue ankle equinus contracture. Clin Podiatr Med Surg 2008;25(4):571–85, vii-viii.
18. Aronow MS, Diaz-Doran V, Sullivan RJ, et al. The effect of triceps surae contracture force on plantar foot pressure distribution. Foot Ankle Int 2006;27(1): 43–52.

19. Kay RM, Rethlefsen SA, Ryan JA, et al. Outcome of gastrocnemius recession and tendo-Achilles lengthening in ambulatory children with cerebral palsy. J Pediatr Orthop B 2004;13(2):92–8.
20. Vulpius O, Stoffel A. Tenotomie der end schnen der mm. Gastrocnemius el soleus mittels mittels rutschenlassen nach Vulpius. In: Orthopadische Operationslehre. Stuttgart (Germany): Ferdinard Enke; 1913. p. 29–31.
21. Silfverskiöld N. Reduction of the uncrossed two-joints muscles of the leg to one-joint muscles in spastic conditions. Acta Chir Scand 1924;56:315–30.
22. Strayer LM Jr. Recession of the gastrocnemius; an operation to relieve spastic contracture of the calf muscles. J Bone Joint Surg Am 1950;32(3):671–6.
23. Baker LD. A rational approach to the surgical needs of the cerebral palsy patient. J Bone Joint Surg Am 1956;38(2):313–23.
24. Lamm BM, Paley D, Herzenberg JE. Gastrocnemius soleus recession: a simpler, more limited approach. J Am Podiatr Med Assoc 2005;95(1):18–25.
25. Tashjian RZ, Appel AJ, Banerjee R, et al. Endoscopic gastrocnemius recession: evaluation in a cadaver model. Foot Ankle Int 2003;24(8):607–13.
26. Saxena A, Widtfeldt A. Endoscopic gastrocnemius recession: preliminary report on 18 cases. J Foot Ankle Surg 2004;43(5):302–6.
27. Baumann JU, Koch HG. Lengthening of the anterior aponeurosis of the gastrocnemius muscle. Operat Orthop Traumatol 1989;1:254.
28. Blitz NM, Rush SM. The gastrocnemius intramuscular aponeurotic recession: a simplified method of gastrocnemius recession. J Foot Ankle Surg 2007;46(2): 133–8.
29. Blitz NM, Eliot DJ. Anatomical aspects of the gastrocnemius aponeurosis and its insertion: a cadaveric study. J Foot Ankle Surg 2007;46(2):101–8.
30. Blitz NM, Eliot DJ. Anatomical aspects of the gastrocnemius aponeurosis and its muscular bound portion: a cadaveric study-part II. J Foot Ankle Surg 2008;47(6): 533–40.
31. Hamilton GA, Ford LA, Perez H, et al. Salvage of the neuropathic foot by using bone resection and tendon balancing: a retrospective review of 10 patients. J Foot Ankle Surg 2005;44(1):37–43.
32. Dayer R, Assal M. Chronic diabetic ulcers under the first metatarsal head treated by staged tendon balancing: a prospective cohort study. J Bone Joint Surg Br 2009;91(4):487–93.
33. Greenhagen RM, Johnson AR, Peterson MC, et al. Gastrocnemius recession as an alternative to tendoAchillis lengthening for relief of forefoot pressure in a patient with peripheral neuropathy: a case report and description of a technical modification. J Foot Ankle Surg 2010;49(2):159. e9–13.
34. Rush SM, Ford LA, Hamilton GA. Morbidity associated with high gastrocnemius recession: retrospective review of 126 cases. J Foot Ankle Surg 2006;45(3): 156–60.
35. Batista F, Nery C, Pinzur M, et al. Achilles tendinopathy in diabetes mellitus. Foot Ankle Int 2008;29(5):498–501.
36. Rao SR, Saltzman CL, Wilken J, et al. Increased passive ankle stiffness and reduced dorsiflexion range of motion in individuals with diabetes mellitus. Foot Ankle Int 2006;27(8):617–22.
37. Naito M, Ogata K. The blood supply of the tendon with a paratenon. An experimental study using hydrogen washout technique. Hand 1983;15(1):9–14.
38. Yosipovitch Z, Sheskin J. Subcutaneous Achilles tenotomy in the treatment of perforating ulcer of the foot in leprosy. Int J Lepr Other Mycobact Dis 1971; 39(2):631–2.

39. Armstrong DG, Stacpoole-Shea S, Nguyen H, et al. Lengthening of the Achilles tendon in diabetic patients who are at high risk for ulceration of the foot. J Bone Joint Surg Am 1999;81(4):535–8.
40. Salsich GB, Mueller MJ, Hastings MK, et al. Effect of Achilles tendon lengthening on ankle muscle performance in people with diabetes mellitus and a neuropathic plantar ulcer. Phys Ther 2005;85(1):34–43.
41. Chilvers M, Malicky ES, Anderson JG, et al. Heel overload associated with heel cord insufficiency. Foot Ankle Int 2007;28(6):687–9.
42. Lin SS, Lee TH, Wapner KL. Plantar forefoot ulceration with equinus deformity of the ankle in diabetic patients: the effect of tendo-Achilles lengthening and total contact casting. Orthopedics 1996;19(5):465–75.
43. Mohsen Allam A. Impact of Achilles tendon lengthening (ATL) on the diabetic plantar forefoot ulceration. Egypt J Plast Reconstr Surg 2006;30(1):43–8.
44. Cevera JJ, Bolton LL, Kerstein MD. Options for diabetic patients with chronic heel ulcers. J Diabetes Complications 1997;11(6):358–66.
45. Holstein P, Lohmann M, Bitsch M, et al. Achilles tendon lengthening, the panacea for plantar forefoot ulceration? Diabetes Metab Res Rev 2004;20(Suppl 1): S37–40.
46. Lagergren C, Lindholm A. Vascular distribution in the Achilles tendon; an angiographic and microangiographic study. Acta Chir Scand 1959;116(5–6):491–5.
47. Stauff MP, Kilgore WB, Joyner PW, et al. Functional outcome after percutaneous tendo-Achilles lengthening. Foot Ankle Surg 2010;17(1):29–32.
48. Hodgen JT, Frantz CH. Subcutaneous tenotomy of the Achilles tendon. J Bone Joint Surg Am 1938;20(2):419–23.
49. Dogan A, Kalender AM, Seramet E, et al. Mini-open technique for the Achilles tenotomy in correction of idiopathic clubfoot: a report of 25 cases. J Am Podiatr Med Assoc 2008;98(5):414–7.
50. Dogan A, Korkmaz M, Cengiz N, et al. Biomechanical comparison of Achilles tenotomy and achilloplasty techniques in young rats: an experimental study. J Am Podiatr Med Assoc 2009;99(3):216–22.
51. El-Hawary R, Karol LA, Jeans KA, et al. Gait analysis of children treated for clubfoot with physical therapy or the Ponseti cast technique. J Bone Joint Surg Am 2008;90(7):1508–16.
52. Dobbs MB, Gordon JE, Walton T, et al. Bleeding complications following percutaneous tendoachilles tenotomy in the treatment of clubfoot deformity. J Pediatr Orthop 2004;24(4):353–7.
53. Burghardt RD, Herzenberg JE, Ranade A. Pseudoaneurysm after Ponseti percutaneous Achilles tenotomy: a case report. J Pediatr Orthop 2008;28(3):366–9.

Surgical Reconstruction of the Diabetic Charcot Foot
Internal, External or Combined Fixation?

John J. Stapleton, DPM[a,b,c], Thomas Zgonis, DPM[d,*]

KEYWORDS

- Charcot foot • Diabetes mellitus • Internal fixation • External fixation • Surgery
- Reconstruction

KEY POINTS

- Charcot neuroarthropathy of the foot and ankle is a devastating neuropathic complication that can eventually lead to a lower extremity amputation.
- Most common fixation methods used for the treatment of the diabetic Charcot foot include internal fixation, external fixation, or a combination of both fixations.
- Bone resorption, fragmentation, and osteoporosis increase the technical demands of using internal fixation to address diabetic Charcot foot and ankle deformities.
- External fixation has shown favorable results in diabetic Charcot reconstruction with severe bone loss, osteoporotic bone, postseptic deformity, nonunion, ongoing osteomyelitis, peripheral vascular disease, and poor soft tissue envelope.
- Combined internal and external fixation methods for the diabetic Charcot foot and ankle may be necessary in certain clinical case scenarios.

INTRODUCTION

The causes of Charcot neuroarthropathy (CN) are numerous and multifactorial. As a result, multiple diabetic-related comorbidities are commonly encountered in patients with CN. Careful consideration and management of these comorbidities are important in determining the overall treatment strategies along with fixation methods. The presence of peripheral arterial disease is commonly seen in this diabetic population and many times can be found in the early stages of CN. However, most of the deformities

[a] Foot and Ankle Surgery, VSAS Orthopaedics, 1250 South Cedar Crest Boulevard, Suite # 110, Allentown, PA 18103, USA; [b] Lehigh Valley Hospital, Allentown, 1251 South Cedar Crest Boulevard, Suite # 202A, Allentown, PA 18103, USA; [c] Penn State College of Medicine, Hershey, 500 University Drive, Hershey, PA 17033, USA; [d] Division of Podiatric Medicine and Surgery, Department of Orthopaedic Surgery, The University of Texas Health Science Center at San Antonio, 7703 Floyd Curl Drive–MSC 7776, San Antonio, TX 78229, USA
* Corresponding author.
E-mail address: zgonis@uthscsa.edu

Clin Podiatr Med Surg 29 (2012) 425–433
doi:10.1016/j.cpm.2012.04.003
0891-8422/12/$ – see front matter © 2012 Elsevier Inc. All rights reserved.

podiatric.theclinics.com

associated with CN that are being considered for surgical management are chronic and long-standing. For this reason, patients with CN should be closely evaluated for peripheral vascular disease in any stage of the pathology and before any major reconstruction.

Delayed wound healing and infection are commonly the reasons for surgical failure and subsequent lower extremity amputation in diabetic patients with CN. The presence of immune dysfunction and hyperglycemia results in an impaired inflammatory process that alters the delivery of critical growth factors leading to a negative impact of wound healing. Other causes that could eventually impede wound healing are smoking, morbid obesity, malnutrition, anemia, arterial insufficiency, neuropathy, and nephropathy. A preoperative assessment to address controllable risk factors is important to improve the local environment for favorable wound healing.

Delayed bone healing related to metabolic alterations associated with diabetic fractures and/or CN is also common in this diabetic population. The exact mechanism of diabetic nonunion has yet to be determined, but the neurovascular and autonomic dysfunctions along with inflammatory mediators and metabolic derangements can lead to decreased bone callous formation in the presence of increased osteoclastic activity. The combination of poor diabetic fracture healing along with recurrent or progressive fracture patterns is a common phenomenon in diabetic patients with CN. For this reason, fixation methods must consider the delay in bone healing, decreased bone mineral density, and/or potential for the loss of fixation when reconstructing foot and ankle deformities associated with CN.

TREATMENT GOALS FOR THE DIABETIC CHARCOT FOOT

The ultimate goal of deformity correction in diabetic CN patients is to provide a functional lower extremity that is resistant to ulceration or infection. Diabetic limb salvage in CN patients should lead to improvement of a patient's daily activities of living, provide an ambulatory status with or without bracing, and improve the patient's overall quality of life.[1–5]

Joint realignment and arthrodesis procedures are currently being attempted at the midfoot, rearfoot, and ankle level to address the unstable and severely deformed CN that cannot be appropriately braced. Surgical treatment protocols are evolving primarily due to unsuccessful outcomes associated with minor osseous exostectomies to address unstable midfoot deformities or conservative treatment therapies to address severe rearfoot or ankle deformities.

In addition, maintenance of a stable plantigrade foot may be achieved with prolonged postoperative bracing and accommodative shoe gear to avoid catastrophic postoperative complications that can lead to recurrence of deformity, skin and osseous breakdown, and eventual lower extremity amputation.[6–8]

CLINICAL DECISION MAKING FOR DIABETIC CHARCOT FOOT FIXATION

When evaluating a surgical patient with CN, a thorough history and physical examination are necessary to identify the duration and progression of the deformity. Clinical and radiographic findings are assessed for deformity staging, instability, or presence of reducibility. Further medical imaging such as computed tomography (CT) scan or 3-dimensional CT scan may need to be evaluated to determine the bone stock, fracture patterns, and joint malalignment. Determining the degree of bone loss or infected bone segments that may have to be surgically resected is essential in the preoperative period. Consideration of previous management is also important, especially if failed surgical attempts have been performed.

The clinical decision to recommend surgery for CN is multifactorial and patient-dependent and usually depends on the severity of the deformity with or without an ulceration or infection, presence of instability with or without preulcerative lesions that are not amenable to bracing, and presence of recurrent infections, osteomyelitis, and unsuccessful conservative treatments in the ambulatory patient.

Most common fixation methods used for the treatment of the diabetic Charcot foot include internal fixation, external fixation, and a combination of both fixations.

If the soft tissue envelope permits, internal plate or screw fixation can provide stability while correcting the associated deformities. Internal fixation can be used as compression or bridge plating to stabilize CN bone segments. The use of bone grafts with internal plate fixation can be used to address osseous defects of the midfoot, rearfoot, or ankle to optimize bone healing. External fixation is the least invasive technique and may be considered for patients who have a poor soft tissue envelope, large bone defects, severe deformities, peripheral vascular disease, and a history of previous ulcerations or infections. A multiplane circular external fixator can be used for gradual deformity correction, bone transport, in combination with internal fixation, and as a surgical off-loading device for concomitant soft tissue defects.

Intramedullary (IM) nailing has also been used to address unstable or chronic CN deformities of the rearfoot and ankle joints. In the event of infection, an IM nail should be avoided until infection or osteomyelitis is appropriately treated. Postoperative infected IM nailing in CN patients can be quite challenging and requires an extensive surgical management with local cemented antibiotics and stabilization before a clinical decision can be made to further proceed with revisional IM nailing, internal plate/screw fixation, or external fixation to avoid a potential nidus for recurrent infection.

Internal Fixation

Numerous internal fixation techniques have been described to stabilize osseous segments of CN. Bone resorption, fragmentation, and osteoporosis increase the technical demands of using internal fixation to address deformities associated with CN. Standard internal fixation techniques such as lag screws for interfragmentary compression even with standard plate fixation are often not sufficient to stabilize CN-related fractures or dislocations. Evolving techniques have focused on fixation placement along with the advent of stronger fixation plates and screws. The concept of bridge plating is to extend the fixation both proximally and distally using less affected osseous segments to achieve better screw fixation. A drawback of bridge plating is that otherwise normal joints are sacrificed to improve the stability of these internal fixation constructs. However, this concept has led to the theory of extended joint arthrodesis in CN patients with multiple fractures and dislocations. An arthrodesis is extended to include adjacent joints beyond the zone of injury to improve fixation and deformity correction while attempting to prevent further collapse. Anatomically designed plates by various industries have been developed to provide a more rigid construct to perform such procedures while considering the soft tissue envelope and plate design for deformity correction and mechanical stability.

Plantar plating for midfoot arthrodesis has been described as a technique that provides superior strength by placing the plate along the tension side of the arthrodesis site. The technique has been described to produce reliable arthrodesis of neuropathic midfoot deformities. Plantar plating may be suitable for select rocker-bottom CN midfoot deformities that have a sufficient soft tissue envelope and especially in addressing sagittal plane deformities at the navicular-cuneiform-metatarsal joints. Extending the arthrodesis to include the talo-navicular joint and the remaining tarsal joints with this technique can be quite challenging.

Medial plating techniques may be beneficial to address certain CN midfoot deformities with severe abduction or to provide stability to multiple transverse joints of the midfoot. Plate fixation in this manner is placed on the tension side of the deformity. In addition, plate fixation along the medial column allows the placement of screws to cross multiple cortices of the metatarsal and tarsal bones, improving the screw purchase and overall construct stability. Locking plates create a fixed-angle construct by attaching the screw to the plate. These devices were developed to improve fixation in osteoporotic bone, and careful consideration is needed to determine if adequate bone purchase is achieved, since the screw is rigidly attached to the plate. Other plating systems have combined locking and nonlocking abilities for certain osseous pathologies and anatomic placements.[3,4]

Intramedullary metatarsal screws have also been described for midfoot CN reconstruction. These large diameter screws are inserted through the metatarsal joints and extend across the midfoot into the talus or cuboid. Alternative techniques are to insert long axial screws from the talus or calcaneus into the midfoot or forefoot. The technique involves deformity correction and stabilization by placing guide wires for large cannulated screws, confirming the position of the foot and placement of the fixation under C-arm fluoroscopy. Advantages to this technique include the limited open approach for the fixation while the screws are entirely intraosseous, which limits hardware exposure. Possible complications to this technique may be due to lack of compression of the multiple arthrodesis sites, loss of purchase, hardware failure, and resulting deformity that leads to challenging revisional surgeries.

Plate fixation to stabilize the rearfoot or ankle can be used if the soft tissue envelope permits and the CN deformity if free of any ulceration or infection. Various plates and plating techniques have been described. Blade plate fixation is a fixed angle construct providing superior stability to stabilize rearfoot and ankle arthrodesis. Numerous anatomic rearfoot and ankle plating systems have been developed allowing for compression and the use of locking screws. The use of various nonanatomic plates such as the femoral and humeral plates has also been described. These plates are typically selected because of their rigidity and strength while providing multiple screw options to gain purchase into the calcaneus. Plate placement for ankle and rearfoot arthrodesis is dependent on the plane of deformity, previous surgical reconstruction, soft tissue envelope, and presence of ulceration. Lateral, anterior, and posterior approaches have all been performed. Incision placement must be carefully planned, especially if bone resections and shortening of the lower extremity are being performed, as these can result in significant tension on the surgical incisions. These clinical case scenarios need to be considered in detail before fixation constructs are placed to prevent poor soft tissue closure and postoperative complications (**Fig. 1**).

External Fixation

External fixation for CN has shown favorable results in severe bone loss, osteoporotic bone, postseptic deformity, nonunion, ongoing osteomyelitis, peripheral vascular disease, and poor soft tissue envelope. The benefits of circular external fixators are the ability to correct deformities while simultaneously providing stability and compression to achieve an arthrodesis if required. Often, it is necessary to perform adjunctive osteotomies or joint realignment arthrodesis when using circular external fixation for CN. Circular external fixators provide rigidity and stability of the entire construct through the use of transosseous wires that are not dependent on cortical purchase as seen with the use of half pins in monolateral external fixators. Various circular external fixation constructs can be designed to address the midfoot, rearfoot, and

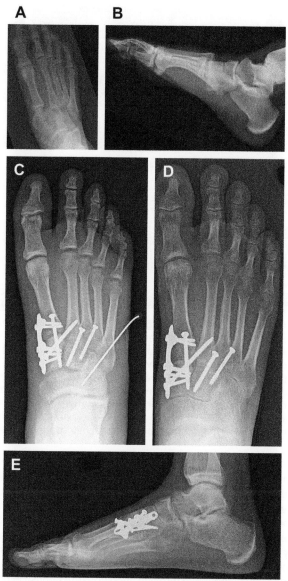

Fig. 1. Preoperative right foot anteroposterior (*A*) and lateral (*B*) radiographic views demonstrating a total homolateral Lisfranc fracture dislocation in a diabetic patient with peripheral neuropathy. Patient underwent a primary tarso–metatarsal arthrodesis of the medial and central columns. Plate fixation of the medial column was used to supplement the interfragmentary screw fixation. The lateral column was stabilized with a Steinmann pin, which was removed at 6 weeks (*C*). Final radiographic (*D, E*) views at 6 months postoperatively, demonstrating successful primary arthrodesis and anatomic alignment of the tarsometatarsal joint.

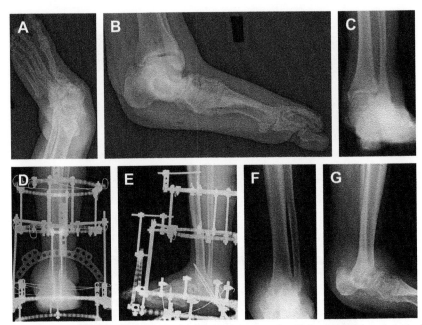

Fig. 2. Preoperative left foot and ankle radiographic views (*A–C*) demonstrating a septic diabetic Charcot rearfoot/ankle with severe peritalar fracture/dislocation. Patient presented with 2 small ulcerations along the medial malleolus and medial aspect of the talonavicular joint. Patient underwent a total talectomy with insertion of antibiotic-impregnated beads and a stabilizing off-loading circular external fixation device for approximately 6 weeks. At that time, the patient had removal of the antibiotic-impregnated beads with a subsequent tibiocalcaneal arthrodesis and circular external fixation (*D, E*). The external fixator was removed at 12 weeks after the definitive arthrodesis was performed. Final radiographic (*F, G*) views at approximately 6 months postoperatively, demonstrating successful arthrodesis and alignment.

ankle CN deformities. The devices are typically characterized as static, stabilization off-loading, or dynamic external fixators depending on the procedures performed.[2–5]

Static circular external fixations devices can be used for primary stability or to augment fixation that was used after joint preparation for arthrodesis procedures. Static circular external fixation constructs are usually prebuilt, allowing ease of application, and they are meticulously positioned to maintain desired alignment of the lower extremity and osseous segments within the zone of injury to promote bone healing. The most common static circular external fixation construct consists of 2 tibia circular rings and a foot plate. This construct can be used to address midfoot, rearfoot, or ankle pathology. Once aligned and stabilized to the lower extremity with multiple transosseous wires or half pins that are placed in anatomic safe zones, additional prebent transosseous wires can be applied to compress selected midfoot or rearfoot joints. Compression of the ankle and the subtalar joint can be accomplished by compressing the foot plate to the tibia circular external fixation.

Stabilization off-loading circular external fixators may vary in design and can be composed of hybrid constructs that incorporate circular rings with a bar to clamp apparatus in aiding to off-load wounds or soft tissue reconstruction. Simple constructs can consist of 1 tibia ring and 1 forefoot ring connected with threaded rods that adequately stabilize and off-load the foot and ankle. Further stability can be achieved

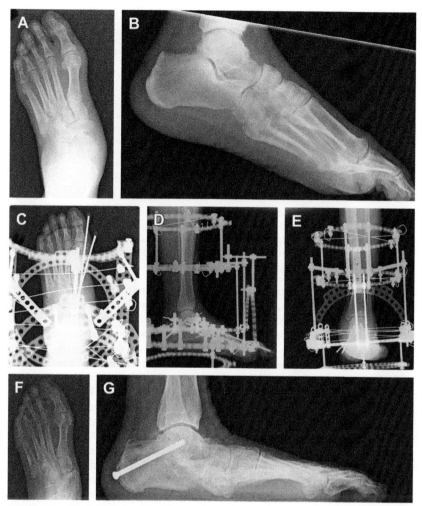

Fig. 3. Preoperative left foot anteroposterior (*A*) and lateral (*B*) radiographic views demonstrating fracture and subluxation at the talonavicular joint and Charcot neuroarthropathy of the rearfoot and ankle. Patient underwent a double arthrodesis of the talonavicular and subtalar joints with the use of internal and circular external fixation to correct the deformity (*C–E*). The circular external fixator was used for internal fixation augmentation and to control the position of the talus within the ankle mortise. The external fixator was removed at 8 weeks postoperatively. Final radiographic views (*F, G*) at approximately 3 years postoperatively demonstrating successful arthrodesis and alignment.

by adding a tibia block that consists of 2 tibia rings connected to a forefoot ring with the possible addition of a transcalcaneal pin. Off-loading constructs that stabilize the rearfoot, ankle, and lower leg are advantageous for providing stability after postseptic debridement of the rearfoot or ankle joint. The external fixator can be used to stabilize the extremity after all necrotic and infected tissue is debrided without the risk of persistent infection. At times, antibiotic-impregnated cement spacers or beads are used to manage the significant bone loss, treat ongoing osteomyelitis, and facilitate healing of future bone grafting. The off-loading external fixation construct that was

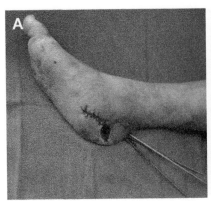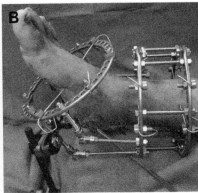

Fig. 4. Example of an open diabetic neuropathic calcaneal avulsion fracture (*A*) that required revisional surgery and fixation with a large diameter internal screw and circular external fixation. Note that the external fixation device allows for appropriate surgical off-loading, stabilization, and local wound for the negative-pressure wound therapy (*B*).

initially applied can later be converted to a static or dynamic circular external fixator to achieve realignment, stability, and compression of the arthrodesis site(s) (**Fig. 2**).

Dynamic circular external fixators are used to address severe long-standing deformities that require gradual progressive deformity correction to obtain joint realignment. These patients are at high risk for neurovascular injury or major soft tissue compromise if correction is performed acutely. The traditional Ilizarov technique and dynamic Taylor spatial frame (TSF) are 2 of the most common methods to achieve gradual correction of multiplane CN foot and ankle deformities. The Ilizarov method typically requires numerous osteotomy and arthrodesis techniques. With a dynamic TSF, the axis of correction can be placed with precision that allows for desired deformity correction. One of the difficulties with correcting severe CN deformities is the possibility of undercorrection or overcorrection when performed with an acute surgical fixation. A dynamic circular external fixator allows continuous postoperative adjustments and fine-tuning of the deformity correction that aid in reducing potential complications of nonunion and malalignment. Another benefit of the previously described techniques relates to improved wound healing, which is extremely important in this patient population. The dynamic nature of the device can facilitate delayed wound closures by reducing tension across pre-existing wounds. Postoperative complications such as pin/wire tract infections and failure, deep infections, malunions, nonunions, and limb loss are possible with these devices. The successful outcome of these techniques is dependent largely on the patient selection, family support, surgical experience, continuous patient education, and overall multidisciplinary team effort to manage the patient's comorbidities and rehabilitation.

Combined Internal and External Fixation

The clinical decision to use combined fixation is to incorporate the major advantages of each technique to provide improved mechanical stability, control adjacent joint mobility, and to protect the soft tissues. Combining internal with external fixation for CN of the foot and ankle needs to be used carefully and with precise surgical planning. The surgical correction of CN midfoot deformities typically involves osteotomies or arthrodesis procedures with internal fixation, and external fixation may be used for controlling and stabilizing the rearfoot, ankle and lower extremity. In addition, when internal fixation is used for a CN midfoot deformity correction, it can be combined with external fixation to address the presence of an equinus contracture associated with the diabetic Charcot foot.[3] Lengthening of the Achilles tendon is debatable and recurrent contracture, overlengthening, and rupture are possible complications. In addition, gastrocnemius recession may improve ankle dorsiflexion but may not improve joint alignment of the ankle or rearfoot in pre-existing severe deformities.

Addressing unstable rearfoot or ankle CN deformities is inherently difficult. The use of incorporating internal with external fixation may be beneficial to realign the osseous segments while providing compression and limited motion to promote an environment favorable to bone healing (**Figs. 3** and **4**). The soft tissue envelope will typically determine the type of plate fixation that can be provided or if an IM is used. Morbid obesity, need for soft tissue protection, adjacent joint immobilization or realignment, and high risk for hardware failure are currently some of the main reasons for combining internal with external fixation for the management of CN deformities.

SUMMARY

Management of CN foot and ankle deformities with respect to fixation choices has not been clearly defined. The surgical team needs to be aware of all available fixation methods and techniques and highly consider their properties and application based on each unique clinical case presentation.

REFERENCES

1. Pinzur MS, Shields N, Trepman E, et al. Current practice patterns in the treatment of Charcot foot. Foot Ankle Int 2000;21(11):916–20.
2. Stapleton JJ, Belczyk R, Zgonis T. Revisional Charcot foot and ankle surgery. Clin Podiatr Med Surg 2009;26:127–39.
3. Capobianco CM, Stapleton JJ, Zgonis T. The role of an extended medial column arthrodesis for Charcot midfoot neuroarthropathy. Diabet Foot Ankle 2010;1. DOI:10.3402/dfa.v1i0.5282.
4. Facaros Z, Ramanujam CL, Stapleton JJ. Combined circular external fixation and open reduction internal fixation with pro-syndesmotic screws for repair of a diabetic ankle fracture. Diabet Foot Ankle 2010;1. DOI:10.3402/dfa.v1i0.5554.
5. Zgonis T, Stapleton JJ, Jeffries LC, et al. Surgical treatment of Charcot neuropathy. AORN J 2008;87:971–90.
6. Saltzman CL, Johnson KA, Goldstein RH, et al. The patellar tendon-bearing brace as treatment for neurotrophic arthropathy: a dynamic force monitoring study. Foot Ankle 1992;13:14–21.
7. Mehta JA, Brown C, Sargeant N. Charcot restraint orthotic walker. Foot Ankle Int 1998;19:619–23.
8. Koller A, Meissner SA, Podella M, et al. Orthotic management of Charcot feet after external fixation surgery. Clin Podiatr Med Surg 2007;24:583–99.

An Overview of Autologous Skin Grafts and Advanced Biologics for the Diabetic Foot

Crystal L. Ramanujam, DPM, MSc, Thomas Zgonis, DPM*

KEYWORDS

- Diabetic neuropathy • Ulcer • Surgery • Skin grafts • Orthobiologics • Diabetic foot

KEY POINTS

- The definitive coverage of acute and chronic diabetic foot wounds is important to reestablish function and prevent infection.
- Autologous skin grafts require a well-perfused granular wound bed that is free of infection typically located at non–weight-bearing aspects of the diabetic foot.
- Advanced biologics can be useful for noninfected deep diabetic wounds, such as those after a partial foot amputation.
- Negative pressure wound therapy can be a useful adjunct treatment modality for either the autologous skin grafts or bioengineered alternative tissues.
- Creative combinations of these techniques may provide innovative approaches for the management of more complicated diabetic foot wounds.

INTRODUCTION

Soft tissue compromise in the diabetic foot can produce a variety of wound types that are induced through several pathways, including traumatic, infectious, neuropathic, and iatrogenic pathways. The definitive coverage of acute and chronic diabetic foot wounds is important to reestablish function and prevent infection. Although diabetes is a multisystem disease that ideally should be controlled in every aspect, the resolution of foot wounds in these patients can pose a significant challenge. Considerations for surgical wound coverage should include the patient's medical status; wound location, type, size, vascularity, and topographic anatomy; function and laxity of adjacent tissue; and the ability of the patient to comply with the demands of proper postoperative care. Adequate surgical debridement, as well as antibiotic therapy when necessary, provides the initial foundation for successful wound coverage procedures. There are a variety of

Division of Podiatric Medicine and Surgery, Department of Orthopaedic Surgery, The University of Texas Health Science Center at San Antonio, 7703 Floyd Curl Drive, San Antonio, Texas 78229, USA
* Corresponding author.
E-mail address: zgonis@uthscsa.edu

Clin Podiatr Med Surg 29 (2012) 435–441
doi:10.1016/j.cpm.2012.04.011
0891-8422/12/$ – see front matter © 2012 Elsevier Inc. All rights reserved.

options on the reconstructive ladder, which can be tailored to address the needs of the wound in question. Autologous split-thickness skin grafts (STSGs) remain a gold standard for the reconstruction of diabetic foot wounds, while orthobiologic skin substitutes have gained increasing attention in recent years by giving surgeons greater flexibility in the treatment of wounds that cannot be addressed with traditional methods. Each of these techniques has unique requirements and ideal clinical settings for optimal outcomes. Furthermore, creative combinations of their use may provide alternate approaches for the management of more complicated diabetic foot wounds.

AUTOLOGOUS STSGs FOR THE DIABETIC FOOT

While the modern meshed skin graft was first described in 1964,[1] the first documented use of skin grafts dates back to 3000 BC in India for soft tissue reconstruction of facial trauma.[2] This technique has evolved through the years to provide a relatively simple, quick, and highly effective method for closure of certain foot wounds.

STSGs require a well-perfused granular wound bed that is free of infection typically located at non–weight-bearing aspects of the diabetic foot. STSGs involve harvesting the epidermis and a variable thickness of the upper layers of the dermis, leaving the remaining layers of dermis to heal by secondary intention.[3] Donor sites may include the thigh or the ipsilateral or contralateral lower extremity of the leg and foot for smaller wounds. Once the recipient wound bed is adequately prepared after sharp manual or mechanical debridement, local hemostasis is achieved and the recipient site is accurately measured. The donor site is usually prepared by local subcutaneous infiltration of 1% lidocaine with epinephrine, and the donor skin is topically prepared with mineral oil. The most common STSG for the diabetic foot has a thickness of 0.018 in and is harvested with an electric dermatome in the length measured for the recipient site. For larger recipient sites, more STSG is harvested with additional passes of the electric dermatome. The harvested STSG is meshed in a 1:1.5 ratio using a commercially available mesher and then secured to the recipient site under minimal tension using skin staples. A bolster dressing or negative pressure wound therapy (NPWT) device can be used to firmly secure the harvested STSG in place during initial incorporation. Weight-bearing status in the postoperative period varies based on the recipient wound location and surgeon's preference (**Fig. 1**).

STSG can be used for a variety of diabetic foot wounds, including acute, chronic, traumatic, surgical, and postamputation wounds. The success in using STSGs over flap donor sites has been reported in patients with diabetes, as well as the use of STSGs over muscle flaps.[4,5] Autologous STSGs are not recommended in wounds with bone, joint, or tendon exposure because these wound beds often lack the local vascularity required for STSG survival.[3]

ADVANCED BIOLOGICS FOR THE DIABETIC FOOT

The first skin substitutes were in the form of xenografts, specifically frog skin used in 1500 BC as described in the Ebers Papyrus.[6] At present, porcine-derived products comprise the most commonly used xenografts and consist of dermis in varying thicknesses from which the epidermis has been removed. Xenografts, such as the OASIS Wound Matrix (Healthpoint Ltd, Fort Worth, TX, USA), are indicated for use in clean partial-thickness wounds and as temporary wound coverages, allowing sloughing with reepithelialization, and reapplication is recommended every 2 to 4 days.[7] A prospective, randomized, controlled multicenter trial by Mostow and colleagues[8] found OASIS to significantly improve the healing of chronic leg ulcers in comparison with treatment with compression therapy alone.

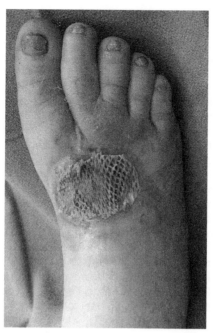

Fig. 1. Autologous STSG for a dorsal granular diabetic foot wound. The patient had a history of an incision and drainage of a dorsal foot abscess.

In 1503, Branca of Sicily first described the clinical use of human skin allografts.[9] Advanced technology has given rise to the development of engineered substitutes using living allograft cells. Apligraf (Graftskin; Organogenesis, Inc, Canton, MA, USA) is a composite allograft comprising bovine type 1 collagen gel and living neonatal fibroblasts as the dermal component, with an epidermal layer composed of neonatal keratinocytes. Veves and colleagues[10] studied the use of Apligraf versus that of control moist gauze dressings, showing complete healing in 56% of the patients in whom Apligraf was used in comparison with 38% in the control group. These allografts can be applied on uninfected partial-thickness or full-thickness diabetic foot wounds. Multiple applications of Apligraf may be needed to achieve complete healing.[10]

In addition, cellular dermal allografts use donor cells to create a regenerative structure seeded with donor fibroblasts that produce components of the extracellular matrix that serve to stimulate the host cells in wound healing. Dermagraft (Advanced Bio Healing, Inc, La Jolla, CA, USA) is one such allograft made from neonatal fibroblasts seeded onto a resorbable polyglactin polymer scaffold. It is indicated for the treatment of chronic diabetic foot wounds without exposed bone, tendon, capsule, or muscle and typically requires multiple applications. A prospective randomized trial by Marston and colleagues[11] showed that 30% of patients who were treated with Dermagraft showed healing compared with 18% of the control patients.

Synthetic bilayer substitutes are acellular products that serve as dermal matrices, which promote ingrowth of host tissues to repair defects. Integra Bilayer Matrix Wound Dressing (Integra LifeSciences Corp, Plainsboro, NJ, USA) is composed of an outer silicone sheet with an underlying bovine collagen and glycosaminoglycan matrix.[12] It is helpful to mesh the Integra Bilayer Matrix Wound Dressing in a 1:1 ratio before it can be secured to the recipient site via bolster or NPWT dressing. The silicone sheet is usually removed at 3 to 4 weeks because vascularization of the matrix has occurred and the neodermis has formed. This biological therapy can also be used for noninfected deep diabetic wounds, such as those after partial foot amputation. Other indications include surgical wounds at flap donor sites that are not ready for STSG. Advantages include its availability, ease of use, and ability to be applied to less-vascularized wound beds. Disadvantages include but are not limited to cost, higher risk for seroma/hematoma formation, rejection, possible reapplication, and potential for infection (**Figs. 2 and 3**).[3]

The GraftJacket (Wright Medical Technology, Inc, LifeCell Corporation for Kinetic Concepts Inc, Arlington, TN, USA) is an alternate acellular dermal allograft indicated for use in lower extremity wounds in patients with diabetes. This product has been processed to remove living cells, preserving an intact matrix that supports repopulation and revascularization by the recipient tissue. Brigido and colleagues[13] demonstrated that a single application of GraftJacket significantly reduced wound size over 4 weeks compared with standard wound care in a study of 40 patients with diabetic wounds.

GammaGraft (Promethean LifeSciences, Inc, Pittsburgh, PA, USA) is an example of a cadaveric human skin allograft that has been irradiated to preserve and sterilize the epidermis and dermis, which adheres to the wound and serves as a vapor barrier, therefore limiting loss of fluids, electrolytes, and proteins. It is indicated for use in partial-thickness and full-thickness chronic wounds and can be stored at room temperature for up to 2 years. Rosales and colleagues[14] reported favorable results when GammaGraft was used for smaller dorsal foot and lower leg wounds.

COMBINED SURGICAL MODALITIES FOR THE DIABETIC FOOT

The relative advantages and disadvantages of the aforementioned options have led to alternative steps and combinations in diabetic wound closure, thereby allowing

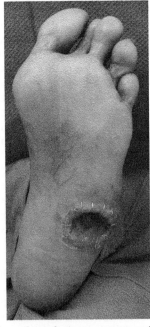

Fig. 2. Advanced biological tissue for soft tissue coverage of a diabetic foot wound on the plantar aspect of the foot.

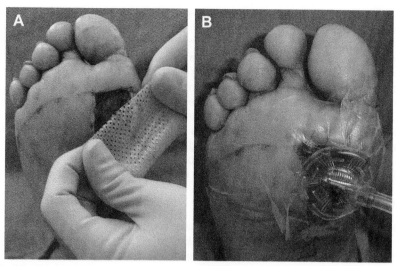

Fig. 3. (*A*) Advanced biological tissue for soft tissue coverage of a diabetic foot wound on the plantar aspect of the foot (*B*) combined with NPWT.

surgeons to navigate the reconstructive ladder with more ease and creativity even in the most difficult of cases. For diabetic wounds that are deep with exposed bone, such as those found after extensive debridement of osteomyelitis, initial treatment with a combination of NPWT and advanced biologics, subsequently followed by

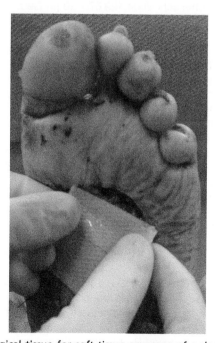

Fig. 4. Advanced biological tissue for soft tissue coverage of a donor site on the plantar aspect of the diabetic foot immediately after the insetting of the local advancement rotational flap.

STSGs, can lead to effective closure of the most complex wounds. This stepwise approach to the coverage of diabetic foot wounds has been shown to decrease inflammatory response and, thereby, decrease hypertrophic scarring, which can result in better function and range of motion of the affected area.[15]

Another clinical scenario, which combines these modalities, is regarding the use of pedicle flaps in diabetic foot reconstruction. Once the flap is raised and inset, the donor site can be temporarily or definitively closed with an advanced biological product. This method is also useful in wounds that require treatment with simultaneous osseous reconstructive procedures since advanced biologics are readily available and can be applied without significantly increasing operative time. If required, STSG can be applied in a staged procedure while harvesting much smaller sized autologous skin, therefore decreasing donor site morbidity (**Fig. 4**).

SUMMARY

Autologous STSG and advanced biologics have each established unique roles in soft tissue reconstruction of the diabetic foot. Before application, the advantages and disadvantages of each of these options need to be carefully weighed along with appropriate patient selection.

REFERENCES

1. Tanner JC, Vandeput J, Olley JF. The meshed skin graft. Plast Reconstr Surg 1964;34:287–90.
2. Baumeister S, Dragu A, Jester A, et al. The role of plastic and reconstructive surgery within an interdisciplinary treatment concept for diabetic ulcers of the foot. Dtsch Med Wochenschr 2004;129:676–80 [in German].
3. Shores JT, Gabriel A, Gupta S. Skin substitutes and alternatives: a review. Adv Skin Wound Care 2007;20:493–508.
4. Zgonis T, Stapleton JJ, Rodriguez RH, et al. Plastic surgery reconstruction of the diabetic foot. AORN J 2008;87:951–66.
5. Ramanujam CL, Facaros Z, Zgonis T. Abductor hallucis muscle flap with circular external fixation for Charcot foot osteomyelitis: a case report. Diabet Foot Ankle 2011;2. DOI: 10.3402/dfa.v2i0.6336.
6. Haynes B. The history of burn care. In: Bosivich J, editor. The art and science of burn care. Rockville (MD): Aspen; 1987. p. 3.
7. Niezgoda JA, Van Gils CC, Frykberg RG, et al. Randomized clinical trial comparing OASIS Wound Matrix to Regranex gel for diabetic ulcers. Adv Skin Wound Care 2005;18:258–66.
8. Mostow EN, Haraway GD, Dalsing M, et al, OASIS Venus Ulcer Study Group. Effectiveness of an extracellular matrix graft (OASIS Wound Matrix) in the treatment of chronic leg ulcers: a randomized clinical trial. J Vasc Surg 2005;41:837–43.
9. Halim AS, Khoo TL, Mohd SJ. Biologic and synthetic skin substitutes: an overview. Indian J Plast Surg 2010;43:S23–8.
10. Veves A, Falanga V, Armstrong DG, et al, Apligraf Diabetic Foot Ulcer Study. Graftskin, a human skin equivalent, is effective in the management of noninfected neuropathic diabetic foot ulcers: a prospective randomized multicenter clinical trial. Diabetes Care 2001;24:290–5.
11. Marston WA, Hanft J, Norwood P, et al. The efficacy and safety of Dermagraft in improving the healing of chronic diabetic foot ulcers: results of a prospective randomized trial. Diabetes Care 2003;26:1701–5.

12. Ramanujam CL, Capobianco CM, Zgonis T. Using a bilayer matrix wound dressing for closure of complicated diabetic foot wounds. J Wound Care 2010; 19:56–60.

13. Brigido SA, Boc SF, Lopez RC. Effective management of major lower extremity wounds using an acellular regenerative tissue matrix: a pilot study. Orthopedics 2004;27(Suppl 1):s145–9.

14. Rosales MA, Bruntz M, Armstrong DG. Gamma-irradiated human skin allograft: a potential treatment modality for lower extremity ulcers. Int Wound J 2004;1: 201–6.

15. Ramanujam CL, Zgonis T. Surgical soft tissue closure of severe diabetic foot infections: a combination of biologics, negative pressure wound therapy, and skin grafting. Clin Podiatr Med Surg 2012;29:143–6.

Current Concepts and Techniques
in Foot and Ankle Surgery

Surgical Treatment Approaches to Second Metatarsophalangeal Joint Pathology

Claire M. Capobianco, DPM, AACFAS

KEYWORDS

- Second metatarsophalangeal joint • Surgery • Freiberg infarction • Arthrodesis
- Arthroplasty

KEY POINTS

- Degenerative causes are the most common in the development of second metatarsophalangeal joint (MTPJ) abnormality.
- Arthroplasty with cheilectomy of the second MTPJ is the most common approach to second MTPJ arthropathy arising from early Freiberg disease or symptomatic gouty arthropathy.
- Interpositional second MTPJ arthroplasty using fat, tendon, or advanced biologics may be used in cases where the second MTPJ is extensively damaged.
- Second MTPJ destructive procedures may include implant arthroplasty or arthrodesis.
- Surgical treatment options for second MTPJ abnormality are etiology dependent and may be joint preserving or destructive in nature.

INTRODUCTION

Although possible, idiopathic, neoplastic,[1] and congenital afflictions of the second and lesser metatarsophalangeal joints (MTPJ) are rare. Degenerative,[2,3] iatrogenic, vascular,[4–9] autoimmune,[10] traumatic,[11] and metabolic[12] causes are predominant, although the extent of articular abnormality may vary widely. Degenerative causes are the most common and include predislocation, subluxation, and dislocation of the second MTPJ resulting in the crossover toe deformity,[13] and chondromalacia resulting from repeated intra-articular corticosteroid injections. The effects of concomitant first ray insufficiency, hallux abductovalgus (HAV) deformity, and aberrant metatarsal parabola are understood as causative factors in the development of the significant portion of second MTPJ abnormality, and the importance of correction of these etiologic factors is assumed.[14] The natural history of the concept of insufficient first ray has been exhaustively described in the literature and are not recapitulated here.

Private Practice, Orthopaedic Associates of Southern Delaware, 17005 Old Orchard Road, Lewes, DE 19958, USA
E-mail address: coatescm@gmail.com

Clin Podiatr Med Surg 29 (2012) 443–449
doi:10.1016/j.cpm.2012.04.004   podiatric.theclinics.com

Vascular insufficiency, another common cause of second MTPJ arthritis, was described by Freiberg in 1914 and is recognized to include a component of microtraumatic injury.[4,6,15] Localized osteonecrosis, flattening of the metatarsal head, and subchondral collapse results from interrupted epiphyseal blood flow. In addition, iatrogenically induced vascular insufficiency and capital osteonecrosis of the second metatarsal head during a metatarsal surgical procedure is possible with overly aggressive dissection.

Similarly, autoimmune and rheumatic causes of lesser MTPJ arthropathy can be devastating. Rheumatoid arthritis may affect the second MTPJ directly with fibular deviation and subluxation, and indirectly as a result of concomitant effects on the first MTPJ. Subluxation and dislocation of the second MTPJ is common with severe rheumatoid HAV deformities and is complicated by concurrent rheumatic articular pannus, tissue atrophy, and frequent ongoing prednisone or disease-modifying antirheumatic drug treatment. Furthermore, the incidence of postoperative infection and wound-healing complications in these patients is not insignificant and cannot be understated.[16]

Infectious causes of second MTPJ pathology are more prevalent in the insensate population, and the pathomechanic imbalances in the insensate foot frequently predispose to plantar ulceration, infection, and contiguous osteomyelitis of the plantar surface of the lesser metatarsal heads.[17] Less frequently, hematogenous spread of distant pathogens has been reported.[18,19] Furthermore, septic arthritis may occur and potentiate serious cartilage damage if not recognized and treated urgently.

Traumatic instances may include crush injury, gunshot injury, and dislocation of the second MTPJ. Crush and gunshot injuries frequently result in massive bone and soft-tissue loss,[11] whereas traumatic dislocations affect soft-tissue collateral structures and vascular supply, and potentiate typical posttraumatic arthritis.[20,21]

Metabolic and endocrine causes of second MTPJ abnormality may result from gout or pseudogout and Charcot neuroarthropathy (CN), although the second MTPJ is infrequently the index site of these conditions. Gout primarily affects the first MTPJ in men and postmenopausal women, but may affect any joint or enthesis. Both crystalline arthropathies primarily potentiate severe inflammation and degeneration of the articular surfaces, and atrophy and tophaceous infiltration of the associated capsule and ligaments.[22] Although CN is incompletely understood, the natural history of the disease and requisite concomitant neuropathy appear to be metabolically driven and predictably result in subchondral sclerosis, cyst formation, and eventual extensive fragmentation and collapse in weight-bearing joints. CN is most commonly seen in the foot at the tarsometatarsal and midtarsal joints, but has been described in the ankle, calcaneus, subtalar joint, and MTPJ. Surgical treatment is not often warranted for forefoot CN, as the extensive degeneration is often masked by dense neuropathy and is asymptomatic. Instead, primarily conservative treatment is indicated.[12,23]

SURGICAL ANATOMY

The vascular supply of the second metatarsal head is primarily through capsular arteries and dorsal, medial, and lateral diaphyseal and metaphyseal arteries arising from the associated dorsal and plantar metatarsal arteries. The intraosseous nutrient artery enters the lateral diaphysis proximally and divides into short proximal and long distal branches that anastomose with the metaphyseal arteries. The joint is innervated primarily through the deep peroneal nerve and the plantar first and second common digital branches of the medial plantar nerve. The associated skin is innervated by the branches of the medial and intermediate dorsal cutaneous nerves.[24]

Medial and lateral collateral ligaments stabilize the joint capsule, and the extensor hood broadens the effective insertion of the long and short extensor tendons to the level of the joint and distally. The deep transverse intermetatarsal ligaments effect static transverse plane stabilization of the joint and the thick, fibrous plantar plate provides dynamic sagittal plane stability.

JOINT-SPARING PROCEDURES
Arthroplasty and Cheilectomy

Arthroplasty and cheilectomy of the second MTPJ is the most common approach to second MTPJ arthropathy arising from early Freiberg disease or symptomatic gouty arthropathy. Resection of affected cartilage and subchondral microfracture or fenestration to facilitate neoangiogenesis is typically performed. Use of adjunctive orthobiologics including collagen matrices and autologous chondrocyte implantation is gaining popularity in ankle and knee arthroplasty, and will likely expand to the small joints in the foot.[25–27] Alternatively, continuous skeletal traction and core decompression[28,29] were published as conservative options for early treatment of Freiberg disease, with the idea that pressure relief and off-loading would halt the osteonecrosis and joint damage, but little follow-up research has been published.

Second MTPJ arthroplasty, with or without orthobiologics, is best for limited involvement of the joint articular surface and is unlikely to be successful in end-stage Freiberg or in isolation in joints with signs of sagittal or transverse plane instability. In these cases, concomitant surgical correction of deformity and deforming forces (via plantar plate repair, adjunctive HAV correction or first tarsometatarsal arthrodesis, selected capsulotomies, and articular stabilization with pinning) is warranted for second MTPJ arthroplasty to be successful long term.

Plantar metatarsal condylectomy is common for treatment of plantar submetatarsal ulcerations with diabetic foot infections when localized osteomyelitis is present. Conversely, if repeated resection is needed or if osteomyelitis is extensive, the entire metatarsal head with or without the affected toe may need to be resected.

Metatarsal Osteotomy

Advanced degenerative changes arising from Freiberg disease may be approached with the dorsiflexory metatarsal osteotomy.[5,7,30] A wedge osteotomy, with the apex located plantarly either intra-articularly[7] or extra-articularly,[5,30] effectively dorsally translates the unaffected native cartilage at the plantar surface of the joint. Typically a 1- to 2-mm wedge is taken, and a single absorbable polyglycolide pin or fully threaded screw is directed from dorsal proximal to plantar distal for fixation. This technique is limited to cases whereby the dorsal one-third of the joint is affected, and also is optimal in a joint that lacks sagittal or transverse plane instability.

Osteochondral Grafting

Osteochondral autologous[31–33] or allogeneic transplant grafting, initially popularized in the knee and ankle, may also be applied to the second MTPJ. Plugs may be harvested from the plantar surface of the talar head, or may be obtained from tissue-bank fresh-frozen cadaver specimens. Joint access is straightforward, and a mosaicplasty approach can address even large defects. Consideration must be given to the inherently small volume of the second metatarsal head and the potential destabilization of the weight-bearing surface with too many plugs. Adjunctive external fixation has also been described in a case study for osteochondral grafting of the second MTPJ.[6] Moreover, cost, availability, and contour profile of the specimens must be considered. Graft subsidence and failure to incorporate are potential pitfalls that would result in large volume loss of the second metatarsal head.

Interpositional Arthroplasty

Interpositional arthroplasty using fat, tendon,[34] or orthobiologic material may be used in cases where the metatarsal head (or phalangeal base) is extensively damaged. Arthroscopic approaches, though uncommon, have been described, and minimize dorsal scarring postoperatively.[35,36] In traumatic or advanced Freiberg disease, interpositional arthroplasty is often used to minimize pain and preserve motion. Local subcutaneous adipose tissue, fascia, or harvested autologous tendon graft may be interposed in the second MTPJ after joint debridement.

JOINT-DESTRUCTIVE PROCEDURES
Implant Arthroplasty

Hemiarthroplasty and total lesser MTPJ replacement implants[37–39] are also options for initial or revisional procedures, although these are considered joint-destructive options. Initially the Swanson implant was used, but periprosthetic fracture and significant synovitis were noted as frequent complications. Periarticular bone void after explantation of these implants was also a concern. The newer-generation metallic implants are of lower profile and require less osseous resection, but have not been widely studied. The joint must be free of infectious agents, and in a postseptic joint scenario, bone biopsy and appropriate cultures are warranted before consideration for hemiarthroplasty or total joint replacement.

Arthrodesis

Arthrodesis of the second MTPJ may ultimately be necessary in cases of severe abnormality or as a salvage attempt after failure of other procedures. Karlock[40] first described fusion of the second MTPJ, and subsequent investigators have advocated fusion with adjunctive autologous grafting, with or without monolateral mini-external fixators, and in conjunction with other forefoot fusions.[41] Steinmann pins, Kirschner wires, screws, or locking plates may be used to fixate the arthrodesis, but inherent difficulties include small area of joint surface and limited approaches for fixation. The ideal angle for fusion has not been formally addressed, although alignment ought to mirror that for the typical first MTPJ arthrodesis in the sagittal plane. Explantation of failed implants or extensive involvement of osteonecrosis may result in significant bony void that requires autografting. In addition, in the severe rheumatoid foot or crossover toe deformity, digital neurovascular embarrassment may occur.

Amputation

Although not often considered first-line therapy, in specific patient populations with severe crossover toe deformity, amputation of the second toe may be an appropriate treatment option. In these cases the patient's morbidities, activity level, age, or personal preference play a critical role in the decision-making process.

SUMMARY

Surgical treatment options for second MTPJ abnormality are etiology dependent and may be joint preserving or destructive in nature. Orthobiologics may be used adjunctively, although research is scarce. The approaches have advantages and disadvantages, with the emphasis always on preservation or reconstruction of stabilizing structures to retain functionality of the second MTPJ. Outcomes studies and comparative studies are needed to compile recommendations for surgical algorithms.

REFERENCES

1. Chiang CH, Jou IM, Wang PH, et al. Synovial osteochondromatosis of the second metatarsophalangeal joint: a case report. J Foot Ankle Surg 2011;50(4):458–61.
2. Coughlin MJ, Schutt SA, Hirose CB, et al. Metatarsophalangeal joint pathology in crossover second toe deformity: a cadaveric study. Foot Ankle Int 2012;33(2): 133–40.
3. Shirzad K, Kiesau CD, DeOrio JK, et al. Lesser toe deformities. J Am Acad Orthop Surg 2011;19(8):505–14.
4. Beito SB, Lavery LA. Freiberg's disease and dislocation of the second metatarsophalangeal joint: etiology and treatment. Clin Podiatr Med Surg 1990;7(4): 619–31.
5. Chao KH, Lee CH, Lin LC. Surgery for symptomatic Freiberg's disease: extraarticular dorsal closing-wedge osteotomy in 13 patients followed for 2-4 years. Acta Orthop Scand 1999;70(5):483–6.
6. DeVries JG, Amiot RA, Cummings P, et al. Freiberg's infraction of the second metatarsal treated with autologous osteochondral transplantation and external fixation. J Foot Ankle Surg 2008;47(6):565–70.
7. Lee SK, Chung MS, Baek GH, et al. Treatment of Freiberg disease with intraarticular dorsal wedge osteotomy and absorbable pin fixation. Foot Ankle Int 2007;28(1):43–8.
8. Mifune Y, Matsumoto T, Mizuno T, et al. Idiopathic osteonecrosis of the second metatarsal head. Clin Imaging 2007;31(6):431–3.
9. Scartozzi G, Schram A, Janigian J. Freiberg's infraction of the second metatarsal head with formation of multiple loose bodies. J Foot Surg 1989;28(3):195–9.
10. Clayton ML, Leidholt JD, Clark W. Arthroplasty of rheumatoid metatarsophalangeal joints. An outcome study. Clin Orthop Relat Res 1997;(340):48–57.
11. Verheyden CN, McLaughlin B, Law C, et al. Through-and-through gunshot wounds to the foot: the "Fearless Fosdick" injury. Ann Plast Surg 2005;55(5): 474–8.
12. Sinacore DR. Acute Charcot arthropathy in patients with diabetes mellitus: healing times by foot location. J Diabetes Complications 1998;12(5):287–93.
13. Yu GV, Judge MS, Hudson JR, et al. Predislocation syndrome. Progressive subluxation/dislocation of the lesser metatarsophalangeal joint. J Am Podiatr Med Assoc 2002;92(4):182–99.
14. Myerson MS, Badekas A. Hypermobility of the first ray. Foot Ankle Clin 2000;5(3): 469–84.
15. Love JN, O'Mara S. Freiberg's disease in the Emergency Department. J Emerg Med 2010;38(4):e23–5.
16. Bibbo C. Wound healing complications and infection following surgery for rheumatoid arthritis. Foot Ankle Clin 2007;12(3):509–24, vii.
17. Newman LG, Waller J, Palestro CJ, et al. Unsuspected osteomyelitis in diabetic foot ulcers. Diagnosis and monitoring by leukocyte scanning with indium in 111 oxyquinoline. JAMA 1991;266(9):1246–51.
18. Muratori F, Pezzillo F, Nizegorodcew T, et al. Tubercular osteomyelitis of the second metatarsal: a case report. J Foot Ankle Surg 2011;50(5):577–9.
19. Yuen MC, Tung WK. An uncommon cause of foot ulcer: tuberculosis osteomyelitis. Emerg Med J 2001;18(2):140–1.

20. Brown TD, Johnston RC, Saltzman CL, et al. Posttraumatic osteoarthritis: a first estimate of incidence, prevalence, and burden of disease. J Orthop Trauma 2006;20(10):739–44.
21. Tadros AM. Fracture-dislocation of the second metatarsophalangeal joint: a case report. J Am Podiatr Med Assoc 2009;99(6):525–8.
22. Roddy E. Revisiting the pathogenesis of podagra: why does gout target the foot? J Foot Ankle Res 2011;4(1):13.
23. Trepman E, Nihal A, Pinzur MS. Current topics review: Charcot neuroarthropathy of the foot and ankle. Foot Ankle Int 2005;26(1):46–63.
24. Sarrafian SK. Anatomy of the foot and ankle. 1st edition. Philadelphia: J. B. Lippincott Company; 1983. p. 294–390.
25. Brigido SA, Troiano M, Schoenhaus H. Biologic resurfacing of the ankle and first metatarsophalangeal joint: case studies with a 2-year follow-up. Clin Podiatr Med Surg 2009;26(4):633–45.
26. Dixon S, Harvey L, Baddour E, et al. Functional outcome of matrix-associated autologous chondrocyte implantation in the ankle. Foot Ankle Int 2011;32(4): 368–74.
27. Koulalis D, Schultz W, Heyden M. Autologous chondrocyte transplantation for osteochondritis dissecans of the talus. Clin Orthop Relat Res 2002;(395): 186–92.
28. Morandi A, Prina A, Verdoni F. The treatment of Kohler's second syndrome by continuous skeletal traction. Ital J Orthop Traumatol 1990;16(3):363–8.
29. Freiberg AA, Freiberg RA. Core decompression as a novel treatment for early Freiberg's infraction of the second metatarsal head. Orthopedics 1995;18(12): 1177–8.
30. Lin SY, Cheng YM, Huang PJ. Freiberg's infraction—treatment with metatarsal neck dorsal closing wedge osteotomy: report of two cases. Kaohsiung J Med Sci 2006;22(11):580–5.
31. Tsuda E, Ishibashi Y, Yamamoto Y, et al. Osteochondral autograft transplantation for advanced stage Freiberg disease in adolescent athletes: a report of 3 cases and surgical procedures. Am J Sports Med 2011;39(11):2470–5.
32. Nagura I, Fujioka H, Kokubu T, et al. Autologous osteochondral plug transplantation for osteochondrosis of the second metatarsal head: a case report. J Med Case Reports 2011;5:308.
33. Miyamoto W, Takao M, Uchio Y, et al. Late-stage Freiberg disease treated by osteochondral plug transplantation: a case series. Foot Ankle Int 2008;29(9): 950–5.
34. Zgonis T, Jolly GP, Kanuck DM. Interpositional free tendon graft for lesser metatarsophalangeal joint arthropathy. J Foot Ankle Surg 2005;44(6):490–2.
35. Maresca G, Adriani E, Falez F, et al. Arthroscopic treatment of bilateral Freiberg's infraction. Arthroscopy 1996;12(1):103–8.
36. Lui TH. Arthroscopic interpositional arthroplasty for Freiberg's disease. Knee Surg Sports Traumatol Arthrosc 2007;15(5):555–9.
37. Shi K, Hayashida K, Owaki H, et al. Replacement of the first metatarsophalangeal joint with a Swanson implant accompanied by open-wedge osteotomy of the first metatarsal bone for hallux valgus in rheumatoid arthritis. Mod Rheumatol 2007; 17(2):110–4.
38. Miller ML, Lenet MD, Sherman M. Surgical treatment of Freiberg's infraction with the use of total joint replacement arthroplasty. J Foot Surg 1984;23(1):35–40.
39. Bordelon RL. Silicone implant for Freiberg's disease. South Med J 1977;70(8): 1002–4.

40. Karlock LG. Second metatarsophalangeal joint fusion: a new technique for cross-over hammertoe deformity. A preliminary report. J Foot Ankle Surg 2003;42(4): 178–82.
41. Jeffries LC, Rodriguez RH, Stapleton JJ, et al. Pan-metatarsophalangeal joint arthrodesis for the severe rheumatoid forefoot deformity. Clin Podiatr Med Surg 2009;26(1):149–57.

Management of Pedal Puncture Wounds

Ronald Belin, DPM[a],*, Scott Carrington, BA[b]

KEYWORDS

- Puncture wound • Foot • Foot infection • Antibiotics

KEY POINTS

- A comprehensive medical and vaccination history is essential for patients presenting with pedal puncture wounds. The timing and location of the puncture wound is important for assessing possible risks and complications.
- Osteomyelitis is a potential complication following a puncture wound. Identification of infectious organisms is imperative to assist in appropriate antimicrobial coverage.
- Treatment and management of pedal puncture wounds may vary among physicians. Puncture wounds should not be treated lightly, significant complications can occur.

Puncture wounds of the foot are a common injury, and infection associated with these injuries may result in considerable morbidity. These wounds may harm underlying structures, introduce foreign bodies, and deposit inoculum that leads to infections. Schwab and Powers[1] reported that patients presenting to the emergency room for puncture wounds showed infection rates of 6% to 11%. The study on wound sites by Patzakis and colleagues[2] indicated that 34 of their 36 inpatients had pyarthrosis, osteomyelitis, or both. For these reasons, when treating patients with puncture wounds it is important to have an efficient approach that is well thought out. Accurate diagnosis, assessment, and management are crucial in preventing a poor prognosis.

CLINICAL PRESENTATION

Children will often present to the emergency room with puncture wounds, particularly barefooted children playing outdoors during warmer months.[3] Haverstock and Grossman[4] also noted that construction workers and laborers are prone to this type of trauma as a result of occupational hazards (**Fig. 1**). Nails are the most frequently seen object in puncture wounds, but other items such as needles, glass, wood, plastic, metal, and even water have been known to cause this type of injury.

Understanding the timing of the injury to presentation is important for treatment protocol. A wound more than 6 hours old has a higher probability of infectious organisms,

[a] Broadlawns Medical Center, 1801 Hickman Road, Des Moines, IA 50314, USA; [b] Des Moines University College of Podiatric Medicine and Surgery, Des Moines, IA, USA
* Corresponding author.
E-mail address: rbelin@Broadlawns.org

Clin Podiatr Med Surg 29 (2012) 451–458
doi:10.1016/j.cpm.2012.01.009
0891-8422/12/$ – see front matter © 2012 Elsevier Inc. All rights reserved.

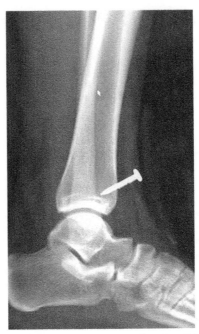

Fig. 1. Lateral radiograph showing a puncture wound to the tibia caused by a roofing nail fired from a nail gun. (*Courtesy of* Broadlawns Medical Center, Des Moines, IA; with permission.)

and after 48 hours there is a greater risk of complications.[5,6] The history should also detail if the patient has made any attempt, successful or not, to debride the wound, to assess the possibility that the foreign body has been broken into pieces or has penetrated deeper.[7]

High-pressure injection injuries, such as those from paint guns and power washers, can often present as puncture wounds. These unique wounds have an increased incidence of oil, paint, or foreign debris deeply embedded within the puncture site. Patients often present with pain and minimal swelling. Because of the nature of these wounds and the increased likelihood of foreign debris being spread along facial planes, high-pressure injection injuries should be considered for surgical intervention.[8]

A comprehensive medical and vaccination history in patients presenting with a puncture wound is essential for proper treatment. Risks of complications are greatly increased in patients with peripheral vascular disease or who are immunocompromised.[9] Special attention should be also paid to patients with diabetes, because of the unique comorbidities that are often present. Diabetic patients are also at an increased risk of developing an infection secondary to trauma.[10] A thorough review of the tetanus immunization history is crucial, as it has been noted that tetanus is 3 times more common and fatalities are 4 times more common among diabetic patients.[11] Often diabetics will have abnormal immune responses to infection. Compromised vascular status and ischemia can decrease the erythema associated with a local infection while simultaneously contributing to the increased degree of infection. Peripheral neuropathy also complicates the risk factors in the diabetic patient. Lavery and colleagues[10] demonstrated that the loss of protective sensation in the lower extremities prolonged the time from injury to treatment because of the "delayed recognition of a limb-threatening problem."

PHYSICAL EXAMINATION

Location of the puncture wound is important for assessing the possible risks and complications. Patzakis and colleagues[2] developed a schematic that can be used to quickly assess the likelihood of infection (**Fig. 2**).

The plantar aspect of the foot was divided into 3 zones. Zone 1 extends from the metatarsal necks to the distal phalanges, zone 2 extends from the distal aspect of the calcaneus to the metatarsal necks, and zone 3 comprises the plantar aspect of the calcaneus. Patzakis and colleagues found that puncture wounds in zone 1 had the highest risk for development of osteomyelitis, followed by zone 3. Zones 1 and 3 are of significance because of the limited soft tissue and underlying osseous structures in these areas. It has also been reported that the most common occurrence of osteomyelitis in children is seen in the calcaneus.[3] Patients with puncture wounds in these locations should be thoroughly evaluated, because of the minimal amount of soft tissue protecting the underlying bony structures.

Conditions of the surrounding tissues should be inspected for foreign matter, debris, and devitalized tissue. It is critical to assess for vascular compromise, and a comprehensive neurologic assessment of the limb should be performed. Range-of-motion testing and function of the surrounding tendons can be helpful in assessing the extent and depth of the wound. Depth of the injury is an important aspect of assessment because more complications are associated with an increased depth of penetration.[2] If examination reveals pain, swelling, erythema, warmth fluctuation, decreased range of motion, and evidence of drainage then infection is indicated, and the wound should be aggressively treated.

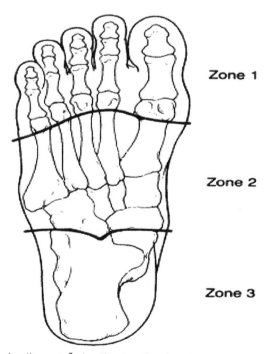

Fig. 2. Patzakis and colleagues'[2] classification for the plantar surface of the foot. (*From* Patzakis M, Wilkens J, Brien W, et al. Wound site as a predictor of complications following deep nail punctures to the foot. West J Med 1989;150:545–7; with permission.)

Local anatomy of the puncture wound is also important for evaluating the extent of the injury, the likelihood of infection, and potential for the foreign body to migrate. Firth and colleagues[12] published a case study in which a 45-mm toothpick fragment went undetected and migrated 10 cm along the flexor hallucis longus tendon sheath. Knowing the anatomy will assist in determining potential routes of migration when a foreign body is suspected, but fails to be detected through either debridement or visualization techniques.

WOUND CULTURE AND MICROBIOLOGY

Identification of infectious organisms is essential in appropriately selecting the proper antimicrobial coverage. *Staphylococcus* and *Streptococcus* are part of the normal skin flora, and as a result are the most common gram-positive organisms associated with pedal puncture wounds.[13] Gram-negative organisms that have been associated with puncture wounds include *Klebsiella*, *Escherichia coli*, and *Proteus mirabilis*.[14] Osteomyelitis is most frequently associated with infections caused by *Pseudomonas aeruginosa*.[15] Organisms such as *Aeromonas hydrophila* and *Mycobacterium marinum* have been isolated from puncture wounds occurring in bodies of water.[15] In addition, *Pasteurella multocida* has been associated with dog bites,[16] and *Eikenella corrodens* has been isolated from human bites and puncture wounds from toothpicks.[17,18]

IMAGING

Imaging techniques are useful for locating and identifying foreign objects, and may be necessary for surgical planning.[19] Plain radiographs should be taken for all puncture wounds to evaluate for retention of a foreign body and to assess for any fractures or osseous changes secondary to infection. Fluoroscopy can aid in surgical debridement, and postoperative films should be taken to confirm that the foreign body has been removed.[7] Small pieces of glass, wood, and rubber will often go undetected on plain radiographs. In these instances advanced imaging techniques should be used.

If glass has been identified as the possible offending object, a retained foreign body should be suspected if a patient has a positive perception of glass in the wound.[20] Glass is often radiopaque, but large fragments can be detected on plain radiographs.[21]

Wood is composed of a porous matrix, and as a result can easily go undetected on radiographs. Nyska and colleagues[22] showed that the use of computed tomography (CT) was a viable technique for visualizing wood in deep tissues when plain radiographs are inadequate. Use of sonography has shown excellent results in both visualizing and ruling out wooden foreign bodies.[23] Sonography is also a more cost-effective option than CT, but a proper patient history and familiarity with sonography imaging is necessary for it to be effective.[24]

If there is a suspicion of osteomyelitis if there is a delayed presentation, radionuclide imaging and magnetic resonance imaging can be beneficial.[7,20] Osteomyelitis characteristically takes 10 to 14 days to show osseous changes on plain radiographs whereas Technetium 99m methylene diphosphonate (^{99m}Tc-MDP) bone scans often detect infection within 24 hours. Although highly sensitive, ^{99m}Tc-MDP has low specificity, and radiolabeled leukocytes are more specific for localizing infections.[25,26]

TREATMENT AND MANAGEMENT

Management of plantar puncture wounds is divisive. Varying approaches and protocols for wound cleansing and use of prophylactic antibiotics have been described in the literature. The first priority in treating puncture wounds should be to convert a contaminated wound to a clean wound. Foreign bodies should be located and removed to prevent them from becoming a nidus for infection.

Simple lacerations without suspicion of a retained foreign body presenting within 6 hours of injury can be treated in the clinical setting. The wound should be debrided and can be irrigated with saline solution, thus aiding in cleansing the wound and preventing infection.[27] In cases of delayed presentation, treatment should consist of incision and drainage. Rough and uneven wound edges are likely to necrose and should be incised to smooth and even the margins. Necrotic tissue should be debrided and the wound carefully irrigated. If present, an abscess needs to be completely drained and aggressively irrigated to ensure all purulent discharge is removed. The wound should then be packed and dressed with a dry sterile dressing. The patient should remain non–weight-bearing during recovery.

In wounds showing signs of infection and/or indications of a retained foreign body, it is recommended that surgical debridement be done. It is important to obtain deep wound and tissue cultures in the operating room. Bone cultures should also be obtained if osteomyelitis is suspected. Primary closure is often thought to be contraindicated for these types of injuries. However, a recent literature review failed to show strong evidence against primary closure of wounds that presented within 24 hours of injury.[28] The patient should be strictly monitored for infection and other wound complications to ensure a positive outcome (**Fig. 3**).

Puncture wounds are susceptible to *Clostridium*. *Clostridium tetani* is a gram-positive anaerobe found in, but not limited to, soil and feces. This organism produces an exotoxin that produces muscle spasms. The patient's tetanus immunization status needs always to be considered when treating these injuries. The most recent Centers for Disease Control and Prevention (CDC) recommendations[8] for tetanus prophylaxis in puncture wounds are outlined in **Table 1**. (This table was created by the authors of this article; physicians may need further clarification at the CDC Web site: http://wwwnc.cdc.gov/travel/yellowbook/2012/chapter-3-infectious-diseases-related-to-travel/tetanus.htm).

ANTIBIOTICS

Prophylactic use of antibiotics has been suggested[29] but remains controversial. In general, prophylaxis should be reserved for those wounds that are highly contaminated,

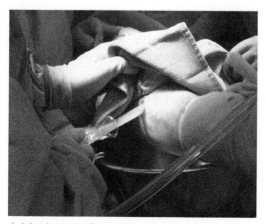

Fig. 3. Irrigation and debridement of puncture wound following removal of nail from the tibia.

Table 1
Centers for Disease Control and Prevention recommendations for tetanus vaccines (DTaP, Td, Tdap) and tetanus immune globulin (TIG) for wound management

Age (y)	History of Tetanus Immunization	Clean, Minor Wounds	All Other Wounds (Puncture Wounds Included)
0–6	Unknown or not up to date on DTaP	DTaP	DTaP and TIG
7–10	Unknown or incomplete DTaP	Tdap and DTaP catch-up dose	Tdap and TIG
11–64	Unknown or <3 doses, or if >5 years since last dose	Tdap	Tdap and TIG
≥65	Unknown or <3 doses	Td or Tdap (if >10 years since last dose)[a]	Td or Tdap[a] (if 5–10 years since last dose)

Abbreviations: DTaP, acellular pertussis vaccine in combination with diphtheria and tetanus toxoids; Td, tetanus-diphtheria vaccine; Tdap, tetanus toxoid, reduced diphtheria toxoid, and acellular pertussis vaccine.

[a] Adults aged ≥65 years who have or who anticipate having close contact with an infant aged <12 months and who have not previously received Tdap should receive a single dose of Tdap to protect against pertussis and reduce the likelihood of transmission; all other adults ≥65 years who have not previously received Tdap may be given a single dose of Tdap instead of Td.

are delayed in their presentation, or occur in at-risk patients. Infections that occur within a couple of days of the injury, are superficial, and are not considered grossly contaminated can be treated with first-generation cephalosporins.[7] For a puncture wound that is at risk for *P aeruginosa*, such as those that occur through shoes,[30] antipseudomonal antibiotics such as ciprofloxacin or levofloxacin may be used. Patients presenting with more significant wounds should be started on empiric antibiotic therapy, which should then be modified according to the culture and susceptibility results. Broad-spectrum coverage is indicated for grossly contaminated wounds and patients at risk for infection, such as diabetics and the immunocompromised. Broad-spectrum coverage may consist of amoxicillin/clavulanic acid, trimethoprim/sulfamethoxazole, or a mix of clindamycin and ciprofloxacin.

SUMMARY

Puncture wounds should be not be treated lightly, so accurate diagnosis and treatment is paramount. The pathophysiology and management of a puncture wound is dependent on the material that punctures the foot, the location and depth of the wound, time to presentation, footwear, and the underlying health status of the patient. Postpuncture wound infections that fail to respond to antibiotics should lead the clinician to suspect the retention of a foreign body. Osteomyelitis caused by *P aeruginosa* remains the most devastating sequela to plantar puncture wounds. If a foreign body is suspected and signs of local infection are present, aggressive treatment should be undertaken. Early incision and drainage, vaccination, and the use of proper antibiotics can lead to positive outcomes and prevent limb-threatening circumstances.

REFERENCES

1. Schwab R, Powers R. Conservative therapy of plantar puncture wounds. J Emerg Med 1995;13:291.

2. Patzakis M, Wilkens J, Brien W, et al. Wound site as a predictor of complications following deep nail punctures to the foot. West J Med 1989;150:545–7.
3. Baldwin G, Colbourne M. Puncture wounds. Pediatr Rev 1999;20:21–3.
4. Haverstock B, Grossman J. Puncture wounds of the foot. Clin Podiatr Med Surg 1999;16(4):583–96.
5. Chisholm C, Schesser J. Plantar puncture wounds: controversies and treatment recommendations. Ann Emerg Med 1989;18:1352–7.
6. McDevitt J, Gillespie M. Managing acute plantar puncture wounds. Emerg Nurse 2008;16(5):30–6.
7. Racz R, Ramanujam C, Zgonis T. Puncture wounds of the foot. Clin Podiatr Med Surg 2010;27:523–34.
8. Bussewitz B, Littrell S, Fulkert K, et al. High-pressure water injection of the foot with associated subcutaneous emphysema: a case report. J Foot Ankle Surg 2010;49:339e16–20.
9. Armstrong DG, Lavery LS, Quebedeaux TL, et al. Surgical morbidity and nondiabetic adults. J Am Podiatr Med Assoc 1997;87:321.
10. Lavery L, Armstrong D, Wunderlich R, et al. Risk factors for foot infections in individuals with diabetes. Diabetes Care 2006;29(6):1288–93.
11. Lavery L, Harkless LB. Infected puncture wounds in the adult with diabetes: risk factors for osteomyelitis. J Foot Ankle Surg 1994;33:561–6.
12. Firth G, Roy A, Moroz P. Foreign body migration along a tendon sheath in the lower extremity. J Bone Joint Surg Am 2011;93:e38 (1–5).
13. Joseph W, LeFrock J. Infections complicating puncture wounds of the foot. J Foot Surg 1987;26:530–2.
14. Miller E, Semian D. Gram-negative osteomyelitis following puncture wounds of the foot. J Bone Joint Surg Am 1975;57:535–7.
15. Joseph WS. Infections following trauma. In: Joseph WS, editor. Handbook of lower extremity infections. 2nd edition. New York: Chruchill Livingstone; 2003. p. 84–90.
16. Lee JL, Buhr AJ. Dog bites and local infections with *Pasteurella septica*. Br Med J 1977;2:169.
17. Bilos Z, Kucharchuk A, Metzger W. *Eikenella corrodens* in human bites. Clin Orthop 1978;134:320–4.
18. Imoisili MA, Bonwi AM, Bulas DI. Toothpick puncture injuries of the foot in children. Pediatr Infect Dis J 2004;23:80–2.
19. Lau LS, Bin G, Jaovisidua S, et al. Cost-effectiveness of magnetic resonance imaging in diagnosing *Pseudomonas aeruginosa* infection and after a puncture wound. J Foot Ankle Surg 1997;36:36–43.
20. Steele M, Tran L, Watson W, et al. Retained glass foreign bodies in wounds: predictive value of wound characteristics, patient perception, and wound exploration. Am J Emerg Med 1998;16(7):627–30.
21. Courter BJ. Radiographic screening for glass foreign bodies: what does a negative foreign body series really mean? Ann Emerg Med 1990;19:997–1000.
22. Nyska M, Pomeranz S, Porat S. The advantage of computerized tomography in locating a foreign body in the foot. J Trauma 1986;26:93–5.
23. Rockett MS, Gentile SC, Gudas CJ, et al. The use of ultrasonography for the detection of retained foreign bodies in the foot. J Foot Ankle Surg 1995;34:478–84.
24. Peterson J, Bancroft L, Kransdorf M. Wooded foreign bodies: imaging appearance. AJR Am J Roentgenol 2002;178:557–62.
25. Blume PA, Dey HM, Daley LJ, et al. Diagnosis of pedal osteomyelitis with Tc-99HMPAO labeled leukocytes. J Foot Ankle Surg 1997;36:120–6.

26. Palestro CJ, Love C. Nuclear medicine and diabetic foot infections. Semin Nucl Med 2009;39:52–65.
27. Fernandez R, Griffiths R. Water for wound cleansing. Cochrane Database Syst Rev 2008;231:CD003861.
28. Eliya M, Banda G. Primary closure versus delayed closure for non bite traumatic wounds within 24 hours post injury. Cochrane Database Syst Rev 2011;91: CD008574.
29. Pennycook A, Makower R, O'Donnell A. Puncture wounds of the foot: can infective complications be avoided? J R Soc Med 1994;8:581–3.
30. Rubin G, Chezar A, Raz R, et al. Nail puncture wound through rubber-soled shoe: a retrospective study of 96 adult patients. J Foot Ankle Surg 2010;49:421–5.

Index

Note: Page numbers of article titles are in **boldface** type.

Clin Podiatr Med Surg 29 (2012) 459–464
doi:10.1016/S0891-8422(12)00087-0
0891-8422/12/$ – see front matter © 2012 Elsevier Inc. All rights reserved.

podiatric.theclinics.com

Moving?

Make sure your subscription moves with you!

To notify us of your new address, find your **Clinics Account Number** (located on your mailing label above your name), and contact customer service at:

Email: journalscustomerservice-usa@elsevier.com

800-654-2452 (subscribers in the U.S. & Canada)
314-447-8871 (subscribers outside of the U.S. & Canada)

Fax number: 314-447-8029

Elsevier Health Sciences Division
Subscription Customer Service
3251 Riverport Lane
Maryland Heights, MO 63043

*To ensure uninterrupted delivery of your subscription,
please notify us at least 4 weeks in advance of move.

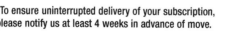

Printed and bound by CPI Group (UK) Ltd, Croydon, CR0 4YY

03/10/2024

01040445-0020